# Healing the Unaffirmed

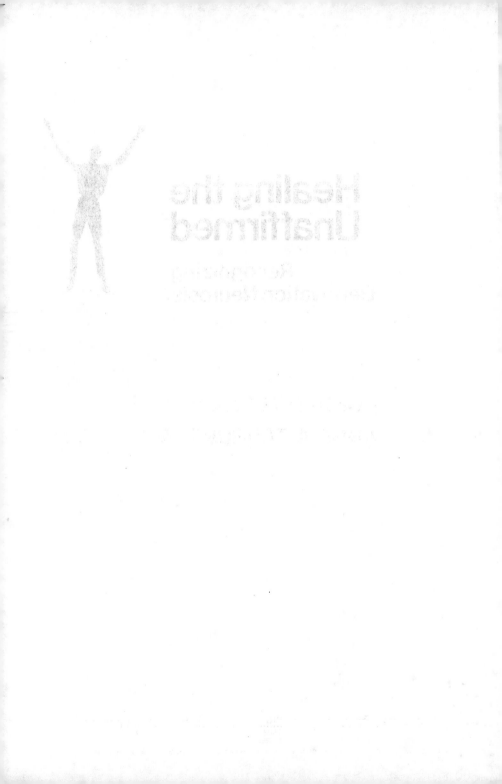

# Healing the Unaffirmed

## Recognizing Deprivation Neurosis

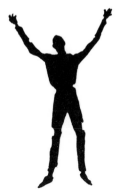

**CONRAD W. BAARS, M.D.**

**ANNA A. TERRUWE, M.D.**

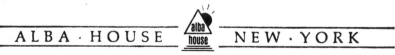

ALBA · HOUSE   NEW · YORK

SOCIETY OF ST. PAUL, 2187 VICTORY BLVD., STATEN ISLAND, NEW YORK 10314

A revised and shortened version of *Loving and Curing the Neurotic* (New Rochelle, N.Y.: Arlington House, 1972).

_____ *Library of Congress Cataloging in Publication Data*

Baars, Conrad W
 Healing the unaffirmed.

   A rev. and abridged version of the authors' Loving and curing the neurotic, published in 1972.
   Includes bibliographical references.
   1. Neuroses. 2. Parental deprivation. I. Terruwe, Anna Alberdina Antoinette, joint author. II. Terruwe, Anna Alberdina Antoinette: Loving and curing the neurotic. III. Title.

RC530.B3          616.8'5          76-7897
ISBN 0-8189-0329-5

*Designed, printed and bound in the United States of America by the Fathers and Brothers of the Society of St. Paul, 2187 Victory Boulevard, Staten Island, New York, 10314, as part of their communications apostolate.*

# AUTHORS' PREFACE

Since the days of Sigmund Freud, the words "neurosis" and "repression" have been practically synonymous, and for good reason. The mechanism of repression has been recognized by psychiatrists everywhere as being at the root of every known neurosis. But even though therapies aimed at uncovering of repressed material have brought cure or relief to countless neurotics, every psychiatrist has encountered a certain number of patients who did not respond significantly. Some patients, in fact, became worse as therapy continued. As existing therapies were found wanting, new ones were researched and tested until they met with the same fate as far as these intractable neurotics were concerned. At certain times the patients were accused of failing to cooperate in the therapeutic process, at other times the personalities of the therapists bore the brunt of the blame.

The possibility that the neurosis in these patients was not caused by repression, and therefore could not possibly respond to uncovering techniques, never received serious attention from the psychiatric profession. This remained so even when psychiatry became acquainted with the *maternal deprivation syndrome,* and the deprivation of the child's fundamental need for love and affection was considered to be only an aggravation of a later neurosis caused by repression, or perhaps as a predisposing factor in the development of such a neurosis.

Our clinical experience did not differ from that of the psychiatric profession in general when our own particular vision of the nature of repressive neurosis brought about unusually gratifying therapeutic successes, especially in obsessive-compulsive neurotics. We also encountered many neurotics whose illnesses did not in the least respond to our therapeutic endeavors. It was only by accident that we were alerted to the possibility of non-repressive factors being the sole cause of a neurosis. This type of neurosis, we discovered, appeared to lack certain features which could normally be expected in neurotic patients, and simultaneously presented such unmistakable characteristics of its own that it had to be distinguished from the classical repressive neurosis. Since this syndrome results from the frustration or deprivation of the natural sensitive need for affirmation in the infant, baby, or growing child by the mother, father, or both, we have given it the name *frustration* or *deprivation neurosis*.[1] Its cure requires, of course, a therapeutic approach essentially different from that indicated for repressive neuroses.

Of course, we do not claim that the symptoms of the deprivation neurosis, described in the following chapter, represent something new or original in themselves. However, what is original and new—and, more importantly, eminently practical—is the grouping of these symptoms into a syndrome separate from, though often associated with, a classical freudian neurosis. Unless therapists learn to recognize the factual distinction between two essentially different types of neurosis—the listing of the deprivation neurosis in the Diagnostic and Statistical Manual of Mental Disorders is long overdue—it will be very difficult if not impossible for unaffirmed people to receive the most effective therapy.

Support for this contention comes from at least two sources. First from the growing realization in the psychiatric profession that "appropriate diagnostic labels are lacking for a certain number of neurotic patients and that traditional exploratory psychotherapy is ineffective in this new kind of neurotic caseload for whom the unconscious seems to have lost most of its mysterious and noxious quality."[2]

Second, from the scores of inquiries received from inadequately or totally unaffirmed persons who recognized themselves without difficulty in reading *Loving and Curing the Neurotic*. By far the largest percentage of them stated that they had been in psychiatric therapy for years to no avail and that they had never felt that their suffering was really understood by their therapists. Merely realizing from reading our book that their suffering made sense and that there were some persons who understood their dis-ease, was a great relief and a source of hope in many of these people. These tragic testimonials to the as yet incomplete body of knowledge of our relatively young specialty will, we hope, be a powerful challenge to all therapists of neurotic individuals.

Our own observations during a combined total of 60 years of clinical practice confirm those described in the psychiatric literature which point to the ever-growing caseload of patients with neurotic and neurotic-like symptomatology. In our opinion this is the result of an alarming increase of the number of deprivation neurotic patients (or, if their clinical symptoms are less pronounced, inadequately affirmed persons) together with a gradual decline in that of persons with a classical, repressive neurosis. Therefore, we would like to disseminate the description of this neurosis and its treatment in a quicker and more economical manner than is possible through the expensive 500-page original edition. This need is even more pertinent and urgent in view of the fact that it is not only the psychiatric and allied professions which must be engaged in the treatment of inadequately affirmed and deprived neurotic people, but also, and in a way primarily, the non-professional, the man in the street, who must do his share in the prevention and relieving of this particular type of emotional illness. Therefore, we are grateful to Alba House for enabling us to share with non-professionals and professionals alike our knowledge of this new psychiatric syndrome, and of affirmation as the key to all human happiness, by means of an abridged, less costly version.

A few discussions in this abridged version of *Loving and Curing the Neurotic* will be more easily understood when the reader realizes that the original edition also dealt with the neuroses shown by Freud to be caused by the mechanism of repression. We explained why his interpretation of the action of this important mechanism is unacceptable in theory as well as in clinical practice. Moreover, we pinpointed the reason for the generally poor results obtained by psychoanalysis in the treatment of obsessive-compulsive neurotics. Starting with a psychology of normal man—rooted in the *authentic* Christian anthropology of Thomas Aquinas—we built constructively upon the groundwork laid by Freud and showed how a force other than the superego brings about repression. Several case histories were presented in order to illustrate how lasting cures of severe obsessive-compulsive neurotics may be obtained without probing of the unconscious and in a relatively short period of time.

Finally, a brief comment is in order concerning our use of the word "healing" in the title of this book. As psychiatrists and as Christians we are not satisfied with merely restoring our patients to their former level of useful functioning in society. This trend is seen most strongly in social psychiatry according to a quote by Norman Q. Brill,[3] "I expect psychiatry will sooner or later follow the military in the second element of social psychiatry, that is, in shifting the focus from the individual's needs to the needs of society. The individual's effectiveness in fulfilling his responsibility to the needs of the society will become the goal of treatment—not his happiness nor even his safety especially—as we move more and more to a strong centralized government and as the clear distinctions between states of war and peace become less and less discernible."

We want to go beyond solely utilitarian criteria of vocational performance or adjustment in business or profession, and assist our patients in attaining a level of happiness commensurate with their innate capacities and potentialities. This generally involves a greater sensitivity for and keener intellectual appreciation of what is true, good, and beautiful; a greater capacity to love and enjoy; a lesser emphasis on utilitarian pursuits with a decided tempering of the utilitarian emotions[4]; and a greater harmony of interaction between sensory and intellectual life. It is by means of this more balanced and properly weighted inner life that our patients are led to attain the happiness for which they have been created—a happiness which requires an act of the intellect, but also, and most emphatically, a ready responsiveness on the part of the emotional life in the stricter sense of the word, namely, the emotions of the pleasure appetite.

What we mean precisely by this is set forth in detail in the pages which follow.

Conrad W. Baars, M.D. and
Anna A. Terruwe, M.D.

1—In the original edition of *Loving and Curing the Neurotic* we solely employed the term "frustration neurosis." However, it has become clear that for a majority of people the word "deprivation" more so than the word "frustration", connotes a significant, traumatic happening inflicted by the environment on an infant or child. For this reason we have decided to use the term "deprivation neurosis" in the English vernacular, while retaining "frustration neurosis" for use in the Dutch.

2—Paul Chodoff, M.D., "Changing Styles in the Neuroses," read at the 1972 annual convention of the American Psychiatric Association.

3—Professor of Psychiatry, University of California Medical School, in *Psychiatry Digest*, May 1, 1971.

4—Fear, courage, hope, anger, despair. The emotions of the pleasure appetite, in rational or Thomistic psychology, are: love, hate, desire, aversion, joy, sadness.

# CONTENTS

# Healing the
# Unaffirmed

# CHAPTER I

# WHY SO MANY NEUROTICS FAIL TO RESPOND TO PSYCHIATRIC TREATMENT

Before describing the type of neurosis which we have called deprivation neurosis, we want to explain *why* and *how* we arrived at the diagnosis of this particular syndrome.

From time to time in our private practice of psychiatry we saw individuals who, in spite of manifesting typical neurotic symptomatology, appeared to lack certain symptoms which one would normally expect in such patients. For example, we observed people who were seriously disturbed emotionally but whose morbid fear—unmistakable as it was in their entire attitude—did not seem to have a repressive action on their other emotions. This observation struck us as being contrary to what is generally accepted as characteristic of every fear or anxiety neurosis. At the same time we were at a loss to explain why our particular therapeutic approach—derived from our Christian anthropologic view of man—which had proven so successful in most obsessive-compulsive neurotics, did not have the desired effect in those other emotionally disturbed people.

Although these and other puzzling observations intrigued us continuously, their solution escaped us until one day our eyes were suddenly opened as a result of a remark by one of our patients, a twenty-five year old girl with a doctorate in physics and mathematics. In spite of her high degree of intelligence, she possessed an unusually infantile emotional life. One of the main symptoms for which she had consulted us was an intense anxiety.

Although our provisional diagnosis had been anxiety neurosis, our efforts to discover the repressive mechanism had remained futile. After several months of psychotherapy had gone by without any noticeable sign of progress, she remarked one day, "Doctor, nothing that you say has any effect on me. For six months I have been sitting here hoping you would take me to your heart . . . you have been blind to my needs."

These words came as a revelation to us. Evidently this patient, whose mother had been an extremely cold and businesslike woman, felt like a child. She needed only one thing—namely, to be treated in a tender, motherly fashion. We had always realized that a cold, impersonal mother-child relationship, like the one existing in this case, could be a predisposing factor for a classical neurosis by generating such an all-pervading feeling of fear that emotional conflicts would readily lead to deep repressions. We began to ask ourselves whether this circumstance—the lack of motherly love and tenderness—by itself would be sufficient to bring about a neurotic illness without the further action of a repressive process.

Once this thought had occurred to us, we began to observe more and more patients whose history and clinical symptomatology confirmed our hypothesis that the mere fact that a child is frustrated in its natural need for love, tenderness, and unconditional acceptance, is sufficient to produce a neurosis which—as far as its symptoms are concerned—is essentially different from neuroses caused by repression. At the same time we came to realize why we had been unsuccessful in treating these patients. Until then our treatment of obsessive-compulsive neurotics had been directed at the elimination of a repression, and therefore could not be expected to correct the underlying cause of this type of neurosis. This neurosis obviously would require its own particular therapeutic approach.

Some time after we had arrived at these conclusions and had worked them out in more detail, we became acquainted with the work of the psychoanalytic author, Germain Guex, who described an almost similar clinical syndrome in her *La névrose d'abandon.*[1] On the third page of this work Guex states that in a number of her cases, classical analysis—described as "gradual exploration of the unconscious for the purpose of discovering the well-known complexes (whether Oedipal, castration, sadistic, or anal . . .)"—has proved to be ineffective. These are cases in which the patient has not yet arrived at an Oedipus situation and no repression has taken place. Instead, there exists, according to Guex, a state of emotional desertion which should be cured in a "less impersonal and more humane fashion" than is typical of classical analysis.

Guex calls these cases "*névrose d'abandon*," a term taken from Dr. Charles Odier's *L'angoisse et la pensée magique.*[2] According to Odier, the *abandonment neurosis* develops when a child is abandoned in the first years of his or her life. This may be a real or merely an imagined abandonment. Odier sees this type of neurosis particularly, in fact, almost exclusively, in cases of imagined abandonment: "An abandoned individual, therefore, is someone who feels or believes himself to be abandoned without good reason." While Odier's "*névrose d'abandon*" contains a more hysterical element, this is not true of Guex's understanding of this syndrome. Her concept is based on a real abandonment and is, therefore, much more closely related to our deprivation neurosis.

Our own thinking in this matter is based on the fact that man is a growing, changing, and developing creature in every aspect of his being, including his emotional life. His emotional life evolves only gradually from infancy until adulthood. Progressing from one stage to the next, it can do so only if the lower stage has reached its full development through adequate gratification of its natural needs. This gratification is absolutely necessary for entering into the next higher stage of emotional development. No phase of growth can be skipped, for only the satisfactory completion and perfection of one phase disposes automatically for the evolution of the next one. It is as Werner says: "Every stage, even the most primitive one, is a relatively closed entity, a life of its own. . ."[3] The baby's psychic needs must be gratified. Its feelings must grow and develop during the first few years of life to such an extent that it will be able to experience the further differentiation of its emotional life during the ensuing childhood years. The child, in turn, must have had the chance to feel and live as a child if he is to be fit to experience fully the disintegration and reintegration of puberty. The adolescent, on his part, cannot attain normal adulthood unless he has had the opportunity to be an adolescent.

It is well known that one of the consequences of repression is psychic retardation. Certain feelings specific for a particular stage of life are prevented from developing by repression, with the result that the emotional life cannot unfold further and remains fixed at that stage. The very same thing may happen without repression, namely, when external circumstances deprive the emotional life of the child from its proper and necessary gratification. Whenever this happens, the child's emotions continue to search restlessly for the gratifications that are rightfully his, and without which the progression to a higher stage of maturity becomes an impossibility. The most telling example is seen when a mother does not give her baby the love which it so desperately needs for its psychic well-being. For that baby's emotional life is doomed to retain a deep-seated dissatisfaction and unrest, a feeling of frustration or deprivation which, involving as it does its most primitive and fundamental striving, affects the child's entire psychic being and distorts its growth.

It is not absolutely necessary that this deprivation take place during infancy for it to have such radical effects. Like the baby, the child also must be given the opportunity to receive the various emotional gratifications proper to his age. If not, his emotional life will show a gap, which prevents further harmonious emotional growth. It is evident that the later in life the deprivation occurs, the fewer these defects will be. For as the emotional life becomes more and more differentiated with the passage of years, the consequences of deprivation will become proportionately less drastic. But when the non-gratification of natural psychic needs affects the very core of his being, as is true in the infant, there develops an emotional illness which to a certain extent resembles classical freudian neurosis, but at the same time presents such unmistakable characteristics of its own that it must be distinguished from the repressive neuroses. We call this syndrome deprivation neurosis, since it results from the deprivation of natural sensitive needs.

The first brief description of our observations of this syndrome appeared in our book, *The Neurosis in the Light of Rational Psychology*.[4] In the present book we shall describe in much more detail the symptomatology of the deprivation neurosis as it involves the emotional life, cognitive life, behavior, and physical condition of the patient. We also will present the various aspects of affirmation therapy. Several case histories are included in an attempt further to clarify our ideas. These ideas pertain, of course, also to the person whose emotional difficulties have not attained the intensity typical of the deprivation neurotic. For sake of convenience we call this person whose emotional troubles are often marked, at least in part, by somatic complaints, or his attempts at self-affirmation, an *unaffirmed* or *inadequately affirmed person.*

1—*La névrose d'abandon* (Paris: Presses Universitaires de France, 1950).

2—*L'angoisse et la pensée magique. Essai d'analyse psychogénetique appliquée à la phobie et la névrose d'abandon* (Neufchatel-Paris: Delachaux & Niestle, 1948).

3—Heinz Werner, *Einführung in die Entwicklungspsychologie*, 4th ed. (Munich: Barth, 1959): "Jede such noch so primitive Stage ist ein relative abgeschlossenes, eigen lebendiges. . ."

4—Anna A. Terruwe, M.D., translated by Conrad W. Baars, M.D.; P. J. Kenedy & Sons, New York, 1960.

# CHAPTER II

# A DEPRIVATION NEUROTIC, OR A FREUDIAN NEUROTIC?

The syndrome of the deprivation neurosis consists of a retardation of the emotional life which is not due to repression. The symptoms which result from this retardation are described in this chapter. The next chapter describes those symptoms which attest to the absence of a repressive process.

## 1. *Abnormal Emotional Rapport with Others*

Persons with a deprivation neurosis find it impossible to establish normal emotional rapport with others. The fact that their emotional life has not sufficiently developed is the cause of a far-reaching influence on their relationships with other people.

This is not so strange when we realize how pronounced the difference is between the emotional life of a child and that of an adult. The baby experiences its contact with another human being only insofar as the latter directs himself to the baby, and to the extent that this contact has significance for the baby's own well-being. Even in the later years of childhood this fact remains one of the most prominent characteristics of the child's emotional life. The emotional life of the adult, on the other hand, has outgrown this egocentricity. He is able to direct his feelings toward another person and to experience the good of the other as his own good. This is the earmark of true, adult love: to be happy with the well-being of another person, because one senses it to be one's own.

Therefore, if an adult has never grown beyond the childhood stage of emotional development, he *is and feels like a child* in his contact with others. As far as his feelings are concerned, he is unable to step outside of himself, but instead remains self-centered, egocentric. Emotionally his contact with others is entirely different from their contact with him. Normally every individual expresses his own feelings in some way or other—in his words, actions, face, gestures, silence and so on; this is inherent in the normal mature way of living. At the same time he considers it a matter of course that others do the same. He also reacts to their feelings with his own, in his own individual manner, thereby remaining himself no matter whether the others are sympathetic or not. In his turn he expects the same of others; he wants a response from them that stems from their true feelings. This essentially is the nature of the contact between two mature, independent human beings.

Persons with a deprivation neurosis, however, are absolutely incapable of establishing such spontaneous contact. They can only establish emotional rapport with another when and to the extent that the other directs himself to them, precisely as a parent orients himself to his child. As long as somebody does this, they feel at ease, safe, and happy; but in every other kind of contact they feel strange and uncertain. When another person leads his own life and expresses his feelings without considering theirs, they feel excluded, left out, outsiders.

It hardly needs to be said that ordinarily people are not as considerate of the feelings of others as deprivation neurotics would like them to be. People lead their own lives with their own interests and goals. It is virtually impossible for them to consider constantly the immature feelings of others. Sometimes, in special cases and under exceptional circumstances this might be possible. This happened in the case of one of our patients, a married woman who, soon after being married, began to manifest the symptoms of a severe deprivation neurosis. (Before her marriage she had been able to maintain her composure by sheer force of will.) Fortunately for her she was married to a man whose love for her knew no bounds and who was able to understand the nature of her illness when this was explained to him. With unparalleled devotion he adjusted himself to her feelings, and thus enabled them to grow slowly and gradually to maturity. But such cases are, as we said before, exceptions rather than the rule. And even in this case it was impossible for the woman to have normal rapport with others who did not understand her and were not as much concerned with her as her husband. In that respect her case was typical of all deprivation neurotics, for they are neither understood nor accepted. They are expected to show normal emotional reactions and to have feelings that are proper to their age. But as these are always lacking, people do not understand them, and consider them strange and different. Unwittingly, others withdraw from them so that they are left alone, abandoned to their fate. They are not accepted because when they show their real feelings, they are considered childish, abnormal, or silly. They are expected to be like others of their own age, more grown-up, more realistic. But, again, that is exactly what they cannot be.

On their part, deprivation neurotics do not understand adults. They consider it a matter of course that the adult relative, friend, or acquaintance should direct himself to them and adjust himself to their feelings. This is as natural for them as it is for a child. And when the adult does not orient himself to them, they experience this as a shortcoming in the other—they feel that he is lacking in love. Reasoning this out for themselves, as they usually do, they feel more and more alone and isolated from others.

### WILLED RAPPORT

In the meantime, being physically and intellectually full grown, they must establish at least some semblance of rapport—superficial though it may be—with others if they are to maintain their position in society. As they cannot do this with their feelings, their only chance to establish such rapport is to do it with their will. To some extent, this can be done. Such a relationship is, of course, not spontaneous, since it does not originate in their innermost feeling selves, as it should, but is consciously willed and therefore superficial. They attempt to establish this contact because they realize the practical need for it. How successful they will be depends to a large measure on their constitution, education, and upbringing. At times they are exceptionally successful, so much so in fact that everything looks normal on the surface. Yet, relationships established in this manner do not satisfy them, for the feelings of friendship and comraderie are meaningless and incomprehensible to them. They maintain such relationships for their practical usefulness, not because they have an inner desire and need to be with another person. One of these patients made the remark once that he had never been able to discover what others meant when they talked about joy or to imagine the feelings of friendship and intimacy. When he was in the company of others at a party or celebration, he never felt anything of what they obviously enjoyed. All he tried to do on such occasions was to keep the conversation going and to make it as interesting as possible for the rest of the group.

Conversely, those who are less energetic by nature have the greatest difficulty—if they succeed at all—in establishing the necessary relationships by means of their will. *In a group they feel like strangers,* and to make conversation is extremely difficult for them. Usually they become so fearful that they withdraw from the rest of the group and stay by themselves. They know they should have contact with others. But to achieve this by sheer will is experienced by them as an encroachment of their freedom. Deprivation neurotic patients have told us repeatedly that when they have willed this contact with another person, they feel as if they had been deprived of something. What they mean is that they have been robbed of their emotional freedom. At no time was it ever their desire to establish contact in this way.

Not all deprivation neurotics realize that their situation is an abnormal one. There are some who hardly care about this lack of emotional gratification. Prominent among these are persons who are successful in establishing their external relationships by means of the will. At the same time there are some who do feel the need for emotional rapport with others. They realize that they lack it, yet they consider their own feelings normal and those of others strange and incomprehensible. This is not difficult to understand, for the only emotional experiences they know are their own. Some of these patients, however, suspect that there is something wrong with them and even arrive at mistaken conclusions about their suspected shortcomings. A good example is the case of a man who told us that he had become aware of a need to have others direct themselves to him in the sense of being especially considerate of him. Since he did not think this to be a normal attitude for a man, he had come to the conclusion that he possessed a feminine emotional life and therefore should have been a woman, as it is natural for a woman to expect a man to show her some special attention and courtesies.[1] We were able to put his mind at ease in this regard by explaining his condition as typical of a deprivation neurosis.

### FRIENDSHIP

The fact that deprivation neurotics are not capable of having normal emotional rapport with adults is at the root of their failure in all relationships in which feelings play a role. Friendship with adults, for instance, is something which they do not really know. Friendship supposes a mutual exchange of feelings, being emotionally tuned in on one another. But this is precisely what is lacking on the part of the deprivation neurotic, and the other person seldom fails to sense this lack even when the deprivation neurotic sincerely tries to will feelings of friendship for the other. Deprivation neurotics may be capable of establishing superficial contacts with acquaintances, even good acquaintances, but these never develop into emotionally satisfying friendships. It is therefore not surprising that all deprivation neurotics say that they feel *lonely*, although not all of them experience this loneliness as a want. Some, in fact, consider it a measure of perfection that they do not need anybody, that they are not bound to any person, and that they are sufficient unto themselves!

MARRIAGE

The feelings of deprivation neurotics fall painfully short in marriage. Marriage is a state of life in which the partners must continuously direct their feelings toward each other and must concern themselves with each other. But this is exactly what the deprivation neurotic partner cannot do; his feelings are gratified only when the other adjusts his feelings to him. This, of course, destroys the proper and normal relationship between married partners. At the beginning of such a marriage, things may sometimes work out quite well. For instance, if the wife is the deprivation neurotic, she may see her husband as more or less of a father figure with whom she can find safety and protection, both qualities which at first may well appeal to the husband's masculine feelings. But after a while the husband cannot but begin to feel a deep dissatisfaction because of the fact that his wife's feelings, instead of going out to him, remain oriented only to herself. Or vice versa: a male deprivation neurotic may seek for motherly tenderness in his wife who, more often than not, will be happy to give this to her husband. Yet, after all, the wife is not the mother but the wife of her husband and, as such, desires the married love in which his feelings are united with hers. Marriages in which one or both partners are deprivation neurotics are therefore *always defective*. Such marriages lack the psychic quality which is essential to every marital relationship, namely, the emotional orientation and surrender to each other. It is for this reason, we believe, that individuals with a severe deprivation neurosis lack matrimonial capacity, and in the years since the publication in the Netherlands of the monograph *De Frustratie Neurose*[2] the Catholic Church has come to recognize deprivation neurosis as an impediment to marriage. It should even be questioned whether the consent given by deprivation neurotics can be considered a truly human act. The following case illustrates this point.

The husband of a former patient of ours, a severe deprivation neurotic, had petitioned his diocesan matrimonial tribunal for an annulment of his marriage. Several years before they were married, his wife had been in therapy for a short time, and then circumstances had made it necessary for her to discontinue her treatment. At that time her emotional life was still in an infantile stage of development. The marriage had been a fiasco from the beginning. This we learned from a member of the tribunal who had been appointed to investigate the validity of the marriage. He had received permission from both partners to obtain a professional opinion as to whether the woman, our former patient, had been free to give her consent to the marriage. The tribunal's representative was informed of our diagnosis at that time and of the chief symptoms of this particular type of neurosis. After having listened attentively, he then read us a letter in which the husband, who had never talked to us or read our writings, listed the same difficulties we had just described as typical of a deprivation neurosis. His foremost complaint was that his wife had been absolutely unable to let her feelings go out to him during the few years they had lived together. This unsolicited confirmation of our diagnosis was for us added evidence that persons with a severe deprivation neurosis should never marry.

#### CHILDREN OF DEPRIVATION NEUROTIC PARENTS

In addition to these difficulties between husband and wife, there are other troubles which concern the children of mothers who are deprivation neurotics. In some cases married women whose emotional lives have remained infantile do not want children at all. One of our patients, a young married woman, simply refused to have a child during the first five years of her marriage, because she felt that she would be unable to cope with the situation if she were to have one. This woman still played with a doll. In this connection it must be mentioned that more than once women with a severe deprivation neurosis have been observed developing a state of disintegration with confusion, fear, and bewilderment following delivery. In all cases this state of disintegration was caused by the woman's realization that she was utterly incapable of what she would have to do shortly, namely, to direct her feelings unselfishly toward her newborn child. The clinician familiar with the syndrome of the deprivation neurosis can do much to prevent the development of a "postpartum psychosis" or to help the unaffirmed woman once it has developed.

When these women have progressed a little further in their emotional development, they usually do want to have a baby. For example, the above-mentioned married woman, who at first still played with a doll, was ready to have a baby after five years of marriage. When the baby came, she was intensely happy. It is most unfortunate, however, that at the same time such women are frequently unable to deal with their older children. They are especially frightened by children who are more assertive and critical. In general, they do best with obedient and affectionate children. One of our patients wanted to have baby after baby, but at the same time sent her older children to boarding schools because she was not able to handle them in a normal, authoritative mother-child relationship.

Another young deprivation neurotic woman wanted her husband to treat her as a mother treats a baby—to hold her, coddle her, and play with her, especially on the weekends when he was home from work. And when she became pregnant for the first time she wished the baby to be a doll, as she was afraid that she would fail completely in trying to take care of a real child. During the early months of her pregnancy she had recurrent dreams in which she forgot to feed the baby and it starved to death. She began to play with dolls during the months before delivery, and was encouraged to do so by us. On her own she switched from oil painting to fingerpainting because "it felt better," and she colored simple coloring books with crayons. As she allowed her emotions to grow freely in this way with our constant encouragement, the symptoms of unreality and confusion, often seen in these patients at such a critical period as a first delivery, did not occur, and she was quite capable of taking care of her little girl without undue tension or anxiety.

### SPIRITUAL ADVISERS

Another state of life in which the incapacity to direct one-self emotionally to others also presents great difficulties is that of spiritual adviser. It is the task of the spiritual adviser, whether priest, minister, or rabbi, to dedicate himself to the spiritual welfare of his fellow men. He can do this work with his will alone, of course, without the participation of his feelings, but in that case his work will bear little or no fruit, for people are moved mainly by feelings; they desire kindness and warm sympathy. To be told in a coldly logical manner what he must do to be saved, or to be helped in a businesslike way in the correction of his faults, has rarely brought a man closer to God. Unfortunately, it is this necessary feeling of sympathy which the deprivation neurotic spiritual adviser lacks. If he is aware of it, and many of them are, his work becomes a burden from which he would rather withdraw.

The case of a priest who suffered from a severe deprivation neurosis demonstrates how intense a burden spiritual work may become. His illness had not been noticed in the seminary because all others there—superiors, spiritual advisers, and professors included—had directed themselves to him and his welfare. This relationship naturally came to an end as soon as he was ordained and had to assume the duties of his state in the parish to which he was assigned. Before long he was unable to carry on with his daily tasks. To visit with his parishioners became sheer torture. He was afraid of giving a sermon; all he could do was to learn something by heart and deliver it without feeling. In the confessional he was never able to establish any personal contact with his penitents. Finally, he could not help but avoid those tasks as much as possible, and he found some relief by occupying himself exclusively with administrative and technical matters.

A Protestant minister in his mid-thirties lasted only a few years in his first assignment in a small parish. He lacked all confidence in himself, was extremely shy and excessively deferential toward his parishioners. He had been too fearful of people to ever ask a girl for a date and considered himself absolutely undesirable as a husband. He had to do his own household chores and cooking as he failed to establish rapport with his parishioners and was utterly unable to sell them on his ideas or needs in the rectory. Although of superior intelligence, he never got his sermon completely prepared for Sunday even after spending the greatest part of the week on it. He lacked all spontaneity; in fact, when he had to go and visit his parishioners he would write down beforehand the prayer he would say and the casual remarks he thought might be appropriate. As a counselor he was a complete failure. He finally withdrew from the ministry and decided to become a librarian, since he loved to read and expected to have only brief, impersonal contacts with people in that occupation.

### TEACHERS

These descriptions are typical of all situations in which feelings play a role. As long as one can deal with others on an impersonal basis, as in the business world, everything is all right, for, in general, business dealings do not require consideration for the feelings of others. Difficulties arise, however, when it is impossible to exclude one's feelings; for instance, in the case of school teachers. Grade school teachers deal with little children who are moved primarily by feelings. In order to get them interested in and desirous of learning, the teacher has to arouse them emotionally. When the children sense the teacher's authority, provided this is a true and mature, not an assumed authority, order is created automatically in their feelings which is then reflected by their orderly behavior in class. The deprivation neurotic teacher, however, does not have this mature feeling and therefore cannot radiate the feelings that produce a desire to be obedient in the children. He lacks order in his class and consequently cannot perform his task. He may then attempt to dominate the children with his will in order to create an orderly atmosphere, but without fail children sense this and the situation usually becomes even worse.

The situation is often somewhat better when the deprivation neurotic teacher has to deal with boys and girls of high school age, for older students already possess more of an intellectual desire to learn. And when he has to teach at a university, the deprivation neurotic encounters practically no difficulties, for at that level of development it is not necessary for his feelings to create the proper atmosphere. We once had a patient, a priest, who found it absolutely impossible to teach young children the catechism, yet he became an excellent professor at a major seminary. He was well aware of his difficulty and once remarked, "Teaching at a seminary is the only thing I can do; I would not be any good in pastoral work." His condition gradually improved during therapy.

Not infrequently these difficulties are so severe that these patients are best advised to give up the teaching profession and to take a job where they have nothing to do with human relations. One of our deprivation neurotic patients was a complete failure as a teacher in grade school, and while on sick leave he decided to work in his brother's music shop. For a while he did well and liked his work, but then began to have difficulties in his relationship with his brother. After changing to an office job and enrolling in a study course, he began to make visible progress in therapy.

If, for some reason, it is impractical for them to abandon the teaching profession, deprivation neurotics may sometimes find that they do better as kindergarten teachers or in teaching of mentally deficient children. In these positions they are more likely to feel certain of their authority and, therefore, are able to have order in their classes. Something similar is seen among deprivation neurotic nurses who as a rule prefer to work on the pediatric floor.

REACTION TYPES

That deprivation neurotic persons may attempt to establish with their wills the rapport which they cannot achieve with their feelings must be further amplified. The manner of their actions and the extent of their success varies considerably with different types of persons. The distinguishing factor in this regard stems from the same difference in constitution and temperament which led us to distinguish between fear neurotics and energy neurotics.[3] There are people who are by nature more inclined to be fearful, and others who tend more toward an energetic and courageous attitude. The former will have a hard time maintaining themselves by their will-power in the face of the difficulties which present themselves to all deprivation neurotics, because the resultant fear readily paralyzes and discourages them.

More energetic patients, on the other hand, are often capable of considerable success in achieving what they want in the world. In fact, it is not at all rare for their emotional retardation to be hidden almost completely behind their successful exterior facade. Still, this does not change the fact that the emotional retardation is present and makes itself felt interiorly. This is well illustrated by the remarks of a forty-year-old scholar, widely known for his erudition and mature judgment, who approached us following a meeting in which we had presented our views on the deprivation neurosis. He was amazed, so he said, to have heard us present such an accurate description of himself, even though we had never known him personally. He told us how he had never enjoyed emotional rapport with other people, and had been able to achieve and maintain his present high status solely by reason of his intellect and will. He had also experienced, and still did at the time, the inner feeling of uncertainty and the other symptoms which we had mentioned during the meeting and which will be discussed in the pages that follow. He was also quite sure that these symptoms had never been noticed by others. He had no trouble understanding what the principal cause of his trouble had been, namely, the particular atmosphere in which he had grown up as a child. His mother had exercised a most domineering role in the family, and had been capable of giving only a token amount of affection to the children. In subsequent psychotherapy this man proved to have a well-balanced personality, a circumstance which explains why, in spite of his deprivation neurosis, he had been able to master the various difficult situations which had occurred in the course of his life.

## 2. Feelings of Uncertainty and Insecurity

Related to this infantile-egocentric aspect of the emotional life of deprivation neurotic persons in their relationships with others is a second symptom—a deep-seated feeling of uncertainty. This feeling has a twofold cause: first of all, their non-affirmation in earliest childhood; and second, the fact that their childish way of feeling makes them unsuited for the adult life they must lead.

In order to feel safe and secure every youthful being needs to be affirmed in his being. A baby is a totally helpless creature; if left to itself, it dies. The baby needs someone who is concerned with its existence, cares for it, and provides it with what it needs. This need is, of course, not a conscious one, for the baby is as yet incapable of any conscious act. Rather, the need is instinctive, for nature never fails to provide what is necessary. Whenever rational guidance is not yet possible, the natural feelings are infallibly directed at providing what is necessary. Just as the baby has an instinctive need for food, so also it needs to experience that it is not alone and is accepted as an existing being. In the beginning it can experience this only by means of the tactile sense, as it is this sense which is the first to develop.

Later on other senses serve this same purpose: the auditory sense by hearing the loving voice, and the visual sense by recognizing its mother's tender look, a look so tender that it responds with a smile. How the salutary feeling of being safe with another person provokes the smile has been expressed beautifully by the Dutch physician-poet, Frederic van Eeden,[4] in his poem, "When Our Baby Smiled for the First Time":

> *"He sent it back to us, our sign of love;*
> *He smiled himself and was alone no more."*

Through all his senses more than in any other way the baby gathers the experience that he is not alone, that others are dedicated to him and care for him. This is the affirmation of its being; the affirmation that complements the fulfillment of its physical needs. It provides the psychic harmony which is the basis for the feeling of inner security upon which his further growth and development becomes possible.

When the child grows older, this feeling of needing help and support does not disappear. His need for people who will provide this help and support remains. And with the development of his intellectual faculty, the instinctive need for certainty that this help will be forthcoming becomes a growing awareness. Indeed, this awareness prompts an ever stronger need for him to experience that he is loved with a love that assures a lasting solicitude and care for him.

When this affirmation as a baby or child is not forthcoming, the child remains in a dissatisfied, frustrated psychic state which involves his entire being and pervades his emotional life with deep-seated feelings of unrest, uncertainty, and insecurity. These feelings remain so deeply buried in his psychic life that they still continue to color his entire emotional life when he becomes an adult. Without doubt, it is this non-affirmation which is the source of the feeling of uncertainty which is found in all deprivation neurotics.

Adding to and feeding on this fundamental feeling of uncertainty is another, the uncertainty caused by the fact that their childish emotional attitude makes them unfit for the adult life they have to lead. They are indeed faced with an extremely difficult task. Physically and intellectually they are grown up. They are regarded as adults and treated accordingly. People expect them to act and react in an adult fashion and do not realize that they are emotionally incapable of doing this. In order to live up to these expectations, the one course of action for them is to do everything willfully, to let reason and will be the sole determinants in deciding what to do. Of course, normal, non-neurotic individuals act in the same will-determined manner, but in their case feelings share in the actions which proceed from the will. This is the reason that normal persons, whose emotions are fully integrated with their intellectual life, have a feeling of certainty when they act. But this certainty is lacking in deprivation neurotics. Even when they are capable of willing certain actions, and reason tells them that they are acting correctly, they lack the corresponding feeling that this is so. This is the source of the uncertainty which they feel with everything they do.

HESITATION AND INDECISIVENESS

All this explains why deprivation neurotic patients always hesitate to act, or, when they have finally brought themselves to act, always change their minds. They find it most difficult to make decisions. As soon as they tend one way, they think of arguments that favor the opposite course of action. We are acquainted with a very intelligent and successful businessman who has not the slightest difficulty in managing his affairs in spite of his deprivation neurosis, for the simple reason that his emotions are not involved in his work. But when something comes up in which he is personally involved—for instance, the purchase of a necktie—he always hesitates a long time before buying one, only to regret it immediately and discard the necktie forever. Another patient, a woman who owns a large shop and runs it most effectively, simply cannot make up her mind when she has to buy birthday presents for her grandchildren. When she goes to the store for this purpose, she is completely at the mercy of the sales clerk. Both patients have this in common—that in their business their decisions are purely rational and matter-of-fact, whereas in other, more personal dealings their feelings play a role which introduces the element of uncertainty and hesitation. Another patient described the same difficulty in a typical manner when she was talking about the purchase of a dress. "As long as the dress is displayed in the window, it is beautiful, but as soon as I have bought it, I begin to doubt whether it is really beautiful!" Displayed in the window, the dress does not concern her personally, but as soon as it is hers, her feelings play a role in her value judgment.

### OVERSENSITIVENESS

Also worth noting is another consequence of this feeling of uncertainty, namely, the fact that the deprivation neurotic is overly sensitive to the opinions of others. One of our patients, for example, bought new living room furniture four times in a five-year period. Each new purchase followed the visit of a relative or friend who failed to show enthusiasm over her furniture, whereupon she began to doubt whether she had made the right choice. This example illustrates the constant need of deprivation neurotics to receive affirmation. They are delighted when a hotel porter or a waiter in a restaurant is kind to them; but when he is a little gruff, they no longer feel at ease and would rather leave the hotel or restaurant at once. When they have performed some external act, they live in continual suspense whether others will approve of it. A preacher finds no rest until he has been reassured that his sermon was excellent. The married woman has a constant need to have her husband tell her she has done a good job cleaning the house, cooking the dinner, or buying shoes for the children. Sometimes such deprivation neurotic women drive their husbands out of their minds by demanding reassurance in everything they do. Usually this is mistaken for vanity on their part, but to call it this is an actual injustice to them, for it is really a manifestation of their own inner uncertainty. A high school teacher with an outstanding record at her school always doubted whether she was doing a satisfactory job and the principal approved of her work. So intense was her feeling of uncertainty that when there was occasionally some minor problem with one of her students, she became overwhelmed with the fear of being dismissed for incompetency.

A significant aspect of the treatment of these patients, therefore, is their constant affirmation by their therapist. Often they have a need to tell the therapist everything they have done and to hear him say that they have done the right thing. This is also the reason why many of these patients send the therapist numerous long letters; needing reassurance in everything, they find it in the fact that the therapist, whom they trust completely, is aware of the things they do.

In view of the preceding, it is not surprising that such patients are very *easily hurt* by critical remarks and slights. When someone disagrees with them or thinks their actions could have been better, they may suddenly become depressed, downhearted, if not bewildered, and unable to carry on their activities. An innocent remark or a constructive suggestion may, in their minds, assume a meaning which the speaker never intended, and is enough to arouse their fundamental feeling of uncertainty and affect everything they do or say. Although they do not dare to disagree or disapprove, they are never completely successful in concealing their feelings of irritation, as the psychomotor aspects of their emotions usually escape their attempts to hide them. Others can usually sense their reactions and then consider them oversensitive in the derogatory sense of the word. These patients always tell us that they do not disagree or disapprove because they *do not want to hurt other people's feelings,* and that they forget about it anyway. But nothing is further from the truth; they do remember each and every time others were not in agreement or seemed critical, and as a result they feel increasingly alone and alienated.

As these patients are motivated primarily by a desire to feel secure with and be liked by others, we explain to them that there are better ways to find this security. Besides the false sense of security which comes from being considered "nice" by everyone, we tell them, there is also a sense of security in knowing who is actually their enemy. And as nobody can ever do or say anything that will please everybody else, what is the sense of trying? To do so anyway, always and everywhere, leads only to frustration and disappointment, if not worse. They are much better off to realize that no matter what they do or say in a group, the basic reaction will always be the same: a certain number will agree, a number will disagree, and again some others will be indifferent. Therefore, if they dare to be themselves with others, they will end up with a number of people liking them for what they do and say, some others disliking them, and a third group totally indifferent to them. Instead of being considered a "nice person" by everybody, as a result of their neurotic way of trying not to hurt anyone and to please everyone, which is actually meaningless, and provides merely a sense of *pseudosecurity*, they will have the security of knowing who their real friends are, and also who dislikes them and therefore cannot be relied on in time of need.

At one time, one of our deprivation neurotic patients was totally upset because he had parked his car in the wrong place and had been told not to do that again in the future. He had been unable to find peace of mind about this incident for three days, and finally became so agitated in brooding about it that he called us for an emergency appointment. Another patient, an attorney in practice for many years, once told us that no day had gone by that he had not thought of the slighting remarks made during hazing in his freshman year at the university!

Closely related to this sensitivity is the observation that some of these patients find it hard to distinguish between remarks made in *earnest* and those made in *jest*. Even when somebody teases them laughingly and obviously with the best intentions, they are plagued by the thought that that person might have been in earnest and really meant what he said![5] One of our patients, a young mother with three children, attempted to take her own life following a remark, made in jest by her husband, that he felt he was pulled between her and the television station where he worked as an engineer.

DESIRE TO PLEASE OTHERS

Still another symptom which stems from this feeling of uncertainty and insecurity is that of always wanting to please others. These patients frequently give the impression of being kind and considerate people, yet their kindness and consideration are determined by their concern to protect themselves from unkind, disapproving, or critical remarks. When we asked one of our patients, a kind and unpretentious man who always went out of his way to please others, his reason for doing this, he replied, "Doctor, it is because I am afraid to lose the other person's love and esteem." Because these people are unable to adapt themselves to others with their feelings, they do so excessively with their will. They are always intent on pleasing others and on avoiding not only what is objectively disagreeable, but also anything which the other person might subjectively experience as unpleasant. Some even go so far that they always want to *give presents* for fear that otherwise the other person would not like them. Some frustration-neurotic teachers worry themselves to death when they have to make out report cards for fear that the parents of their pupils will be displeased and come to school to find fault with them in person. Some deprivation neurotic housewives live in fear of their own servants. One of them, for example, had not dared to give an order for thirteen years, not even such a simple one as "Take this dish to the kitchen"! Sometimes they feel uneasy in a conversation when they have expressed themselves in a negative manner about somebody else. Their concern not to displease others becomes so intense at times that they are afraid not only of being treated unkindly, but even in a kindly fashion. This seemingly *para-doxical anxiety* is a manifestation of their fear that the other has been mistaken in his impression of them and that the next time they meet he will no longer be kind to them!

They are not only afraid of being criticized themselves, but also that others who are closely related to them will meet with criticism. For instance, a young deprivation neurotic girl we know lives in constant fear that her mother will be dressed improperly or say something stupid in a conversation. Another patient always became disturbed when in her opinion her husband did or said something awkward at a party or when they entertained at home.

*Fear of being considered a nuisance* often keeps them from daring to ask for a service from others. How strong this fear may become is well demonstrated in the following case. One of our deprivation neurotic patients shared a hospital room with a man who had lived for years in the tropics as manager of a large rubber plantation and, therefore, was accustomed to giving orders and dealing with employees. One afternoon this man woke up from his nap and rang for the nurse. When she came in, he asked her for the time. The nurse gave him the information requested and left the room again with a smile. Our patient was simply overcome by the fact that his roommate had dared to ring the nurse for such a simple thing as finding out what time it was, and even more that the nurse had responded in such a casual and friendly manner! We also know several deprivation neurotic persons who will never ask someone at the table to pass the salt or pepper for fear of being a nuisance, or who will eat anything in a restaurant no matter whether the food is burned or spoiled.

This symptom, *fear of asking for a favor or service,* is so common that when deprivation neurotic patients have to be admitted to a hospital, we always inform the nurse in charge that they are not allowed to do anything themselves and must be given help with everything. If such precautions are not taken, these patients may take it upon themselves to make their beds and clean their rooms, and may even run errands for other patients!

### HELPLESSNESS

Such patients often feel helpless and ill at ease in company because they are so *self-conscious* and do not know what to do with themselves. When one of our patients, a good-looking and well-dressed woman, has to go to a restaurant, she does not dare to get up and leave for fear that she will make herself ridiculous. A kindergarten teacher died a thousand deaths each time she had to attend a school party: "If I could just sit there without having to say anything, it would not be so bad!" In general, if there is somebody at such a party or gathering who takes an interest in them and draws them into conversation, they are able to manage fairly well, for in that case they feel affirmed. We usually advise these patients to ask questions when in a group since for them this is the least difficult way to establish some contact with others. Another woman patient once told us: "I don't mind thunderstorms, I am not afraid to be alone at home, to make a long trip by myself is no problem at all for me, I was never scared of the air raids during the Nazi occupation during World War II, but when I have to meet people, I am scared stiff!" It may be mentioned that women with deprivation neuroses often are much more at ease with men than with other women, because of the fact that a man directs himself spontaneously to a woman.

These deprivation neurotic individuals are also defenseless in a store when a fast-talking sales clerk tries to make them buy a certain article. They *do not dare to say no*, and buy the article even though they do not want or cannot afford it. For obvious reasons, this often leads to complications when they get home and have to explain their unnecessary or extravagant purchases to their spouses, or figure out what to do with them. Naturally, it would be better if such persons did not go shopping by themselves. The same difficulty also exists for deprivation neurotic housewives who are approached by aggressive door-to-door salesmen. They become easy prey unless the husband, having learned from bitter experience, has made it impossible for his wife to close a sales contract without his signature on the check, or because he does not leave her any ready cash.

Nor is this all. Deprivation neurotics not only go out of their way to please others, but sometimes they try to justify their behavior to themselves. Some do not approve of their exaggerated deference, but experience the reason for it—and properly so—as a fear against which they are utterly helpless. These people react to their behavior—inwardly at least—with rebellion. Others *rationalize* their eagerness to please others and find excuses for doing it. Individuals dedicated to a spiritual life frequently like to consider it a virtue, an act of love of one's neighbor, an act of humility. Naturally, they constantly forget that virtue always holds the middle road between too much and too little, and that in their case there is too much.

### HOARDING

We shall conclude the phenomenology of this emotional uncertainty by reporting one more symptom observed in some deprivation neurotics which, in our opinion, stems from this feeling of uncertainty. We have in mind the need to collect and hoard useless items. One woman patient had several cupboards and four trunks full of all kinds of rubbish: rags, ribbons, string, papers, notebooks, boxes, tags—in short, anything she had ever been able to put her hands on. Like other deprivation neurotics who showed this symptom, she was unable to throw these things away even though there was not the slightest chance she would ever use a single item. We believe that this urge to hoard things stems from the deep-seated feeling of uncertainty and insecurity.

Everything they possess, no matter how small or insignificant, represents a certain security because of the fact that it belongs to them. Patients who manifested this symptom in our practice were all persons who had been totally dependent on others for their existence.

### KLEPTOMANIA

Finally, in a few cases this urge leads to kleptomania. As one patient expressed it: "When I can grab and take something home, I get a greater feeling of security."

### REACTION TYPES

The extent to which this feeling of uncertainty exerts its influence on the personality varies with the person's disposition and temperament. The previously-made distinction between the more energetic and asthenic types also applies here. Those endowed by nature with a more forceful and energetic disposition, aware of their inner uncertainty, force themselves to act as if it did not exist. In this way they are able, although with a certain measure of inner tension, to keep up appearances in the outside world. Yet before long a knowledgeable observer will be able to detect their deep-seated feelings of uncertainty. And what is more, this type of deprivation neurotic always runs the risk of repressing his fears sooner or later, just as camouflaged fear neurotics do.[6] This, of course, may lead to a worsening of their condition, as the repressed fear may grow and spread in all directions. Obviously, the danger of a breakdown always exists, as their way of holding themselves together is an unnatural one which puts an excessive strain on their psychic powers.

The more asthenic, weakly personalities, on the other hand, find it much harder to give themselves an air of self-reliance, and to keep up with others. Usually their feeling of uncertainty will manifest itself much earlier in life in the form of a generalized anxiety, as we have seen in the various cases described in this chapter. There is no end to the ways in which this fear may present itself. We have repeatedly observed—to mention only a few examples—the *fear of hurting others,* of contaminating others when they have a cold, of not daring to learn to drive a car because they are afraid they might injure pedestrians or crash into another car. Some of these patients have been known to feel compelled to remove pebbles or banana peels from the sidewalk to protect others from tripping over them. A most unusual case was that of a wholesale dealer in candy and sweets. He worried himself sick about the possibility of little pieces of glass being hidden among the sweets.

It is not surprising that the first impression given by these patients is that of a fear neurosis, but as we shall explain in Chapter III the fear in the deprivation neurotic is of a different character from that of the fear neurotic.

3. *Feelings of Inferiority and Inadequacy*

Related to their feelings of uncertainty is a third symptom which may be observed regularly in deprivation neurotics; namely, a strong feeling of inferiority and inadequacy. This is to be expected. Their feeling of uncertainty causes them to fail repeatedly in whatever they undertake, and in consequence they develop a sense of being inferior.

FEELING UNLOVED

This manifests itself frequently, particularly in *girls,* in a feeling that nobody loves them and that nobody could possibly love them. The fact that they did not receive love when they were young is later interpreted to mean that they are not worth loving. Moreover, since they are unable to love as adults, they believe that they are devoid of all feelings of love, that they are totally incapable of loving, and that they are not lovable in themselves. They are suspicious of every token of affection, and if somebody is kind to them and cares for them, they continually doubt whether that person really loves them.

A woman with an extremely severe deprivation neurosis lived

amongst people who were all kind and devoted in their unselfish care of her. Yet this woman was absolutely unable to believe that they really loved her, and she reacted to everything that was done for her with indifference and coldness. For, as long as she believed that nobody loved her, all signs of kindness were meaningless and of no value.

Again, other women want to be told continually that they are really loved. Whereas normal adults take it as a matter of course that such a declaration of affection need not be endlessly repeated, these patients consider its relative infrequency as further proof that they are not loved. This reaction, of course, further strengthens their feelings of inferiority. And to make matters worse, they frequently do lose the sympathy of others because of their demanding attitudes. When this happens in a marriage, the result may well be disastrous. Such a deprivation neurotic woman lives in constant fear that her husband does not love her. His slightest failure to pay attention to her, even when it is due solely to the fact that he must attend to his business interests, is enough to make her feel that she does not mean anything to her husband. She may react to this, depending on her temperament, with either a depression or vehement reproaches. In some cases her reaction leads to an intense jealousy which may make life simply unbearable for the husband. Whenever he happens to pay attention to another woman, be it in talking to one at a party, or in giving instructions to his secretary, his wife cannot help but feel that he must love that other woman more than her. This was the case with one of our patients, the wife of a teacher at a high school for girls. It is impossible to describe the many scenes which occurred over and over again because of his teaching assignment. A simple glance at one of the girls, or a remark about one of them, was enough for her to conclude that he liked the girl and not her; she would burst into tears and bitterly reproach him.

The reverse situation may also be seen. For example, we know a man with a severe deprivation neurosis whose wife is really extremely fond of him. He himself is aware of his wife's love for him, and intellectually he is fully convinced that she will never fail him in her love. Yet, in spite of this reasoned certainty, he lives in constant fear that she might become attracted to other men. Although he does his utmost not to show this, the resulting tension under which he lives is felt constantly by his wife and causes her no end of sorrow.

Patients like these often look for reasons why others do not love them. Many girls arrive at the conclusion that they are ugly, or possess a shapeless figure, or lack some desirable feature in their personality. One of our deprivation neurotic patients happened to be a strikingly beautiful girl. One day her mother came to visit us in order to talk about her daughter, and in the course of the conversation we remarked how good-looking her daughter was. To our amazement the mother replied: "Isn't that true, doctor; and what a pity that she thinks of herself as being so ugly!" The fact was that the girl had never told us this; in all her interviews she talked with great difficulty and practically never in reference to herself.

On the other hand, some strikingly beautiful women with a deprivation neurosis were found to rely heavily on their good looks for some measure of feeling confident. They spent considerable time in beauty parlors and spent freely on fashionable clothes in order to find encouragement in admiring looks and compliments. They did this in spite of their prior knowledge that they would have to meet with considerable envy on the part of other women, and with comments of being proud and conceited, if not accusations of wanting to attract other men. The latter was always the farthest thing from their mind, at least as far as intimate affairs were concerned. The feeling of confidence they derived from their good looks and attractive appearance was absolutely necessary to overcome their fear of people, especially when invited to social gatherings. Actually, several of these women felt guilty about their need to rely on their good looks, and considered themselves vain and selfish for spending so much time and attention on themselves. We reassured these women on this point and advised them to continue to rely on their pleasing appearance and thus give others the opportunity to discover also their many other good qualities.

In *boys* the feeling of inferiority frequently manifests itself as a concern over inadequate virility and masculine physique. One of our younger male patients, with an entirely normal physical build, could not rid himself of the idea that as far as masculine development and strength were concerned, he was much inferior to other fellows. On one occasion he compared himself unfavorably with a certain young man whom he described as a really strong and virile fellow. Having accidentally given away the name of this much envied fellow, we could not help being amused, as the latter also happened to be our patient—something which this young man did not know—and not only possessed the same feelings of inferiority, but also envied our young man for the very same physical qualities which the latter envied in him! Finally, young men with a deprivation neurosis sometimes mention feelings of inadequacy with regard to their penis because, in their opinion, it is either too small or too large.

### FEELINGS OF INTELLECTUAL INCOMPETENCE

In men as well as in women, strong feelings of inferiority also occur in relation to intellectual capacity. A medical student of superior intelligence, but with a very severe deprivation neurosis, was absolutely convinced that he would never succeed in his studies. It was only at our insistence that he agreed to take his next examination, but a few weeks later at his regular visit he informed us that he was certain he had failed in all or most of the subjects. As we happened to be personally acquainted with one of his professors, we called him to inquire about the results of this young man's tests. The professor assured us that he had passed them all with excellent marks. When we gave the patient the news, he claimed, however, that it was only because of our friendship with the professor that he had received such good marks, and that he had been allowed to pass only because his teacher felt sorry for him!

A girl with a severe deprivation neurosis always felt that she was incapable of doing anything well, in spite of the fact that she was an unusually gifted person in almost every field. She was of superior intelligence, most artistic, and skillful with her hands. Yet her work was never completed; when she began something, she would give up after a while with the excuse that she "would not be able to finish it, anyway!" However, after a year of treatment, she outgrew her fears and was able to persevere in her efforts. Now she succeeded in everything she undertook. She told us then that she had never wanted to learn before because she feared that if she were to try anything, it would turn out to be a failure. The same symptom is sometimes found in a different form. For instance, several female patients told us that they did not want to wear pretty dresses as children because they were afraid that people would not like them anyway! And if their dresses were old or soiled, at least the clothing could be blamed for the fact that they were not liked!

### REACTION TYPES

The manner in which persons with a deprivation neurosis react to their feelings of inferiority and inadequacy depends—as we have already seen—on their innate temperament. Those with a more asthenic constitution become aggressive, especially toward persons who they know will not hurt them in return. A woman with an extremely incapacitating deprivation neurosis had a husband who loved her dearly and did everything to help and please her. Day or night, every spare moment away from his profession was devoted to his wife. However, when something unpleasant happened to her which she felt she could not endure, she would angrily turn on her husband and blame him for being the cause of all her troubles. She would accuse him of not caring about her, and tell him that he should have known better than to let such a thing happen.

Less asthenic personalities, on the other hand, become depressed. The feeling of not being able to face life weighs heavily upon them and leads to an intense feeling of dejection. This was the case with the medical student we mentioned above. Gradually he lost all courage and was unable to continue his studies. Finally he had to be admitted to a hospital for the mentally ill. Occasionally these states of depression terminate in *suicide* because the person sees no way out of his condition and despairs of ever feeling loved by anyone.[7]

### GUILT FEELINGS

At times these feelings of inferiority and inadequacy give rise to a deep-seated feeling of guilt. When these patients have arrived, intellectually at least, at the level of moral behavior, they attach to their inadequacies an ethical significance which these acts do not possess at all. They see their inability as a fault imputed to the will. They consider themselves evil, devoid of love, without religious feeling, selfish, seeking only themselves, so that as far as they are concerned, every act of theirs cannot fail but confirm their guilt. Because their feelings do not participate in their actions, proceeding as they do solely from the will, they reproach themselves for what they consider false and dishonest actions. As they put it themselves: "I condemn myself for acting differently from what I really feel!"

Such feelings of guilt were also present in a girl who tried to be pleasing to men. She reproached herself for wanting to seduce these men, although actually she was impelled only by her need to be affirmed.

It must be added that these feelings of guilt are very difficult to modify in patients with a deprivation neurosis. They are based on a deep-rooted, virtually ingrained judgment of their own personality. In our experience, however, these feelings of guilt are not found in all deprivation neurotics. In fact, at times they may even be completely lacking. Possibly the role of environment determines to a large extent whether such feelings will be present or not. If too much emphasis in the early years was placed on the obligation to control oneself and avoid sin, such feelings of guilt develop easily because deprivation neurotics—because of their psychic immaturity—are prone to make the judgments of others their own. Also, the presence or absence of an inclination to introspection further determines to what degree such feelings of guilt will manifest themselves in later years.

Many of our patients with intractable guilt feelings have benefited from our advice to meditate on the words of Dr. Carl Jung regarding the need of the psychotherapist *to see and accept himself as he is,* before he can accept his patients as they are. Dr. Jung says:

> To accept oneself as one is may sound like a simple thing, but simple things are always the most difficult things to do. In actual life to be simple and straightforward is an art in itself requiring the greatest discipline, while the question of self-acceptance lies at the root of the moral problem and at the heart of a whole philosophy of life.
>
> Is there ever a doubt in my mind that it is virtuous for me to give alms to the beggar, to forgive him who offends me, yes, even to love my enemy in the name of Christ? No, not once does such a doubt cross my mind, certain as I am that what I have done unto the least of my brethren, I have done unto Christ.
>
> But what if I should discover that the least of all brethren, the poorest of all beggars, the most insolent of all offenders, yes, even the very enemy himself—that these live within me; that I myself stand in need of the alms of my own kindness, that I am to myself the enemy who is to be loved—what then?
>
> Then the whole Christian truth is turned upside down; then there is no longer any question of love and patience; then we say "Raca" to the brother within us; then we condemn and rage against ourselves! For sure, we hide this attitude from the outside world, but this does not alter the fact that we refuse to receive the least among the lowly in ourselves with open arms. And if it had been Christ himself to appear within ourselves in such a contemptible form, we would have denied him a thousand times before the cock crowed even once.[8]

1—Many a modern, "liberated" woman may scoff at this assertion. Yet her efforts to be equal to the man, no matter how successful in terms of society's utilitarian and pragmatic attitudes, do not necessarily disprove the existence of innate, natural inclinations and needs. It is a rather simple matter for a woman to repress or suppress them, and to deny to herself that she is not truly happy when men do not show her that special something commonly reserved for feminine women.

2—Dr. Anna A. Terruwe, J. J. Rowen en Zonen, Roermond, 1962.

3—In speaking about the retarded emotional life of deprivation neurotics, we have in mind the emotional life in its narrower sense; namely, the emotions of the pleasure appetite, such as love, desire, and joy. The emotions of the utility appetite—fear, courage, and anger—are not involved in this retardation, or at least to a much lesser degree. The reason for this difference stems from the fact that the lack of emotional satisfaction, which is the cause of retardation, lies precisely in the pleasure appetite where it exerts its delaying action. Moreover, the influence of the intellect on the emotions of the utility appetite is always much greater than on those of the pleasure appetite, so it is only natural for the development of the emotions of the utility appetite to more readily keep pace with the development of the intellect. The foregoing terms are described and explained fully in the original version of *Loving and Curing the Neurotic.*

4—Dr. Frederik van Eeden (1860-1932), chief literary work: *"De Kleine Johannes."*

5—In this connection it is interesting to note Werner's claim (op. cit., p. 263) that in primitive people and children there is only a thin dividing line between jest and earnest. ("Wir erfahren aus den verschiedensten Gegenden der Welt, wie leicht bei Naturvolkern—ubrigens ganz ähnlich wie bei unseren Kinderen—aus Scherz Ernst zu werden vermag").

6—A camouflaged fear neurotic starts out by repressing an unacceptable emotion through fear. However, not wanting to appear fearful he represses this fear in turn through energy. For a more complete description of this double repression consult the original edition of this book.

7—The most profound psychological insights are often found in the works of poets and dramatists. Taylor Caldwell provides us with a revealing description of a deprivation neurotic in her *Great Lion of God* (Garden City: Doubleday & Co., 1970) when David ben Shebua tells Hillel ben Borush what his father, Shebua ben Abraham, is really like.

"I should ask my father's forgiveness for even suggesting that he is a patriarch. The very idea would revolt him. . . . My father is not what you think he is. He is the creation of the style and postures of others.

He is a mirror of what he believes is admirable. You shattered that mirror. He is now confined to his bed, under sedatives.'

"Hillel was astonished. He said, 'Is it possible I made an impression on him? That I discomfited him? I thought him an armored man, armored in his disdain for such as I.'

" 'You do not understand,' said David. 'My father cannot live without the esteem of others. He cannot endure it that a single man might despise or criticize him. He is not a man. He is an image, easily scratched, easily stained; he is colored plaster.'

"Hillel was even more astonished, but was also incredulous. He said, 'I have heard that of all the traders in Israel, and the merchants, and the bankers, and the stockbrokers, and the investors, he is the most astute! I have heard that in these pursuits he is a man of iron, and cannot be moved.'

" 'That, too, is true,' said David. 'But those he deals with in those matters are men like himself, of sweat and iron and bronze and hard fists. However, only in the reek of the marketplace. It is a different Shebua ben Abraham who returns to his house and goes to his baths and his concubines and his perfumes and his togas. . . . The Shebua ben Abraham who is raucous and adamant in the marketplace is not the Shebua ben Abraham who visits Pilate and King Herod and dines with philosophers and the elegant Greeks. This Shebua is a cosmopolitan, another posture, another appearance, another countenance, another aim, another desire, another aspiration. And that dainty man is easily shattered, easily injured, if others look upon him, even for a moment, as if he is still a man of the marketplace.'

" 'Or a man of flesh and blood,' said Hillel, with bitterness. 'You are implying that I made that delicate man tremble in his plaster and rattled his rings and bracelets? Are you not saying that he is very fragile? Shebua is not one, even in his postures, to care for the opinions of a man like me, who has no pretensions.'

" 'He is fearful of the bad opinion even of a slave,' said David. . . 'I know you have considered me an imitator of him. Let me suggest that he imitates me, instead . . . and that is why he dislikes me'."

8—Free translation from Carl G. Jung, *Die Beziehungen der Psychotherapie zur Seelsorge* (Zurich: Rascher & Cie., 1932).

# CHAPTER III

# A FEAR IS A FEAR, IS A FEAR—OR IS IT?

Retardation of the emotional life, with all the consequences, described in the previous pages, is the first characteristic of deprivation neurosis. A second and equally important characteristic is the fact that this developmental disturbance is not the result of a repressive process. It is true, as a rule, that an infantile emotional life is also seen in repressive neuroses, for the repression makes it impossible for the repressed emotions to mature. Since these emotions remain fixed at an early stage of development, it is not surprising that many of the symptoms described above are also seen in the repressive neuroses, particularly in the fear neurosis. Nevertheless, there are such typical differences between the psychic state of the fear neurotic and that of the deprivation neurotic that one is forced to recognize the deprivation neurosis as a clinical syndrome in its own right.

### LACK OF EXCESSIVE FEAR OR ENERGY

The first difference is that in deprivation neurosis one does not see the most distinctive feature of the repressive neuroses, namely, the hypertrophy of the repressing emotions of fear or energy. In the original edition of this book we explained that a repressive neurosis develops when the emotions of the pleasure appetite, instead of being guided by reason and will, are repressed by an emotion of the utility appetite, whether fear or energy.[1] But such a neurosis develops only when the repressive process has been operating over a number of years. This means that many years of abnormal activity by the repressing emotions causes it to hypertrophy to such an extent that it dominates the entire emotional life of the individual in the form of anxiety or restless striving. It is this hypertrophied fear or energy that is entirely lacking in the deprivation neurosis.

More than once we have treated persons with a very severe deprivation neurosis in whom the only observable symptoms were the infantile emotional life and the accompanying feeling of uncertainty, without a trace of excessive fear or energy. One was a girl of twenty-five, the daughter of prosperous parents, who had never been away from home for studies or employment, as her parents had felt it unnecessary for her to try her hand at anything. Her mother was a strange woman, without feelings for her children, and incapable of giving them, and this girl in particular, any love or affection even when they were infants. Later on we were able to determine that she herself was a deprivation neurotic. As a result of her mother's coldness, the girl's emotional development had been severely retarded; her emotions were typically those of a child. Her only concern was that others would not love her, and for that reason she had built a whole system of fantasies in which she possessed every imaginable quality that would endear her to others. However, there was no trace of a restraining or paralyzing fear. On the contrary, she did exactly as she pleased; in fact, so much so that at one time her conduct necessitated admission to a psychiatric hospital. But she refused to stay there and made her parents take her back home. A tentative diagnosis of schizophrenia was made at that time. A few days later she was brought to us for treatment, and it was not long before we made the diagnosis of deprivation neurosis. Showing no sign of fearfulness or excessive energy, she was filled with but one desire, to be loved. This desire manifested itself in different ways. For example, she directed all her affection at a frequent house guest, a clergyman, who was always kind and good to her. There was no sexual element at all in her affection for this man; she only wanted him to be kind to her. But this desire spurred her on so intensely that she pursued him constantly. He was eventually obliged to órder his house-keeper never to admit to her that he was home. In matters like this, she never showed the slightest restraint. When we were kind to her in treatment, her affection directed itself so intensely at us that it took considerable and constant effort to retain our freedom in the treatment situation. To anticipate an obvious question, we want to state that this girl was neither a psycho-pathic personality nor a hysterical neurotic. As the result of therapy she became a normal young woman fully able to com-plete successfully any task she took upon herself.

DIFFERENCES IN FEAR

Although we have had many more cases like this, the mood of an even greater number of deprivation neurotics is character-ized by pronounced fearfulness. Since this fear stems from deep-seated inner uncertainty, it is of a decidedly different character than the fear of fear neurotics. The latter are always filled with a *fear of something* and try to escape from it in order to be safe. For example, a person is fearful of sexual matters and everything that is related to sex because he has been led to believe that sex is evil and sinful. This fear then makes him avoid and reject everything pertaining to sex; he tries to ban it entirely from his life so that it can never lead to sin.

The situation is completely different in deprivation neurotics. As there is no object that is desired by one emotion and at the same time rejected by another, these patients do not experience an emotional conflict like that of fear neurotics. They fully accept their emotional strivings insofar as such strivings are present. Fear develops only because they do not receive the desired object and thus are continually frustrated. Over the years their fear grows in intensity and scope because these per-sons find it ever more difficult to deal with the varied demands of life. They feel that they cannot cope with life. One might say that their fear is an *existential fear*, not a conative, volitional fear like that experienced by fear neurotics. Their fear is not that they may do something that they should not do or that is forbidden by their moral or social standards, but that they may be faced with certain situations which will prove too much for them. This characteristic of their fear was evident in all the persons we described earlier when we discussed the symptoms of uncertainty.

To put it differently, in fear neurosis the fear is primary and the emotional non-development secondary, while in deprivation neurosis the emotional non-development is primary, and the fear is secondary, the result of this non-development. This also explains why deprivation neurotics do not tend to *cling to their fear*, as fear neurotics do. For the fear neurotic, this attachment is a means of averting an evil, and it takes much effort and persuasion to get them to give it up; they can always think of reasons why it is right to be fearful. In fact, some Catholic patients are almost offended when advised that certain acts of theirs are not formally sinful. A similar attachment is found in energy neurotics, but in terms of their willpower; in some of them it has become an attitude of life that broaches no interference and which they refuse to abandon. But one never sees a deprivation neurotic hold on to his fear in this fashion. For him it is only an evil that he experiences as long as his retarded emotional development makes adjustment to everyday life impossible. But as soon as he achieves this adjustment, the fear disappears by itself.

To differentiate between these two kinds of fear presents a problem only when a repressive neurosis, namely, a fear neurosis, has *superimposed* itself upon a deprivation neurosis. The possibility that these people will be exposed to repression-inducing circumstances is as great as with other people. They are brought up and educated in the same manner and may receive, to mention only this one example, the same premature, fear-inspiring warnings about sin. Moreover, the groundwork for the repressive action from fear usually has been laid already in these people because of their deep-seated feeling of uncertainty, the result of their frustrated affective needs.

*Pseudoneurotic reactions,* or *situational neuroses,* too, develop readily in people with a deprivation neurosis. This is not surprising when we realize that the pseudoneurotic's repressing mechanisms do not stem from inner conflicts, but rather from seemingly insurmountable external difficulties. Situations like these occur only too easily in deprivation neurotics, as they hide the fact that the demands of adult life are too much for them; consequently, nobody protects them from the ordinary stress situations of everyday life which for them become insurmountable obstacles. To arrive at the correct diagnosis is sometimes a difficult matter in these cases. Frequently one will think first of a repressive neurosis, especially as the patients start out by discussing their particular conflicts; only later will it become evident that a deprivation neurosis lies at the root of their difficulties. Experience alone will increase one's capacity to sense the patient's feelings correctly and to evaluate his condition.

### ATTITUDE TOWARDS PLEASURABLE EMOTIONS

Immediately related to the preceding is another characteristic; namely, the entirely different attitude toward pleasurable sensory feelings and emotions on the part of the fear neurotic and the deprivation neurotic. In repressive neurosis, from the beginning, there exists an intrapsychic rejection of certain feelings or desires considered to be harmful. This rejection, caused by stimulation of the utility appetite, has two results: (1) a hypertrophy of the repressing emotion of fear or energy; and (2) as far as the repressed emotion is concerned, an ever deeper rejection. This is the reason that in a repressive neurosis an arising pleasurable desire always provokes an *unconscious inhibition.* The therapy of this kind of neurosis, therefore, is primarily directed at the elimination of these inhibitions; the excessive fear or energy must diminish. Only to the extent that they do diminish is it possible for these pleasurable emotions to be allowed expression. It is not until then that the desires can grow and lead to the enjoyment of a sense good. Until that time it is also impossible for these desires to fall under the dominion of rational control.

The rejection of a sense good is not an issue in the deprivation neurosis. The desire for such a good is not in the least inhibited or blocked, but its attainment is made impossible as a result of external circumstances. In other words, the gratification of the desire is frustrated. Consequently, these patients do not develop an inner rejection of this sense good. The only thing that develops and grows in deprivation neurotics is the persistent activity of the frustrated desire, just as in the repressive neurosis. But, and this is the important difference, this ever more deeply felt frustrated desire grows without activating repressing emotions of fear or energy for the simple reason that there is no repressing emotion. This also explains why these patients, when a change in circumstances makes it possible for this desire to become gratified, are able to give in to it without a sign of unconscious inhibition, and also to enjoy it to the fullest. It is this ability especially that distinguishes this type of neurosis from the repressive kind. *Deprivation neurotics are capable of enjoyment;* much less so are repressive neurotics. In the sex act, for example, the latter experience release of sexual tension but very little actual enjoyment. This, of course, is to be expected. Enjoyment presupposes the ability to yield oneself to the sense good without holding back, but it is precisely this surrender which is inhibited in a repressive neurosis. In deprivation neurosis, however, there is no inhibition, no holding back, and for that reason persons with this type of neurosis experience the full enjoyment of the sense good that is offered to them. To give a very good example: patients who as infants lacked for motherly tenderness, and who later found an individual who was pleased to give them this tenderness, are only too happy to let themselves be treated and coddled as babies. They delight in children's games, in dolls and teddy bears. Grown-up men come to life and find heretofore unknown vitality when they are able to play boys' games.

## REACTION TYPES

As far as this particular reaction to a sense good is concerned, one is able to distinguish, just as with people in general, two types. While all people strive after sense goods, their striving is not always the same in nature. First of all, there are those who become completely fascinated and captivated by the concrete-sensory aspect of an object; these are people endowed with a concupiscible, sensuous nature. There are others who are equally attracted by a sense good, yet whose striving after that sense good has a natural tendency to be ordered and guided by reason. Although not less spontaneous, their striving and desire is more rational by nature.

It is, of course, to be expected that one will find these two types of people among deprivation neurotics. For both types may become exposed to the circumstances which would lead to the development of neurosis. In both, the striving will manifest itself without abnormal inhibitions from fear or emotional energy, yet the manifestation itself will differ in each type. In the former, the sensual element in the striving will be quite pronounced; they show what Odier has called an "affective eagerness, a sentimental gluttony."[2] In the other, this striving expresses itself in a manner that is more calm and balanced.

The sensory desires in the first group have the upper hand, so much so that there is little or no spontaneous concern as to whether or not their desires are reasonable; even moral considerations do not play a role in many cases. We have repeatedly observed that these patients, whenever the opportunity presents itself, do not hesitate to take things that belong to others; they desire these and appropriate them without qualm. They also consider it a matter of course that others are dedicated to them and give them everything they ask. Often it does not even occur to them to show any sign of gratitude. In this respect, their attitude is amoral, but this too is to be expected, considering their infantile level of development.

### FEAR LACKS AN OBJECT

We have come now to the third distinction between deprivation neurosis and repressive neurosis. In the latter there is always an object that brings about the repression and excites the repressing fear or energy. In the course of the development of the neurosis this object may grow and expand until in the most serious cases it virtually comprises the entire sense life. But no matter how much it grows there is always an object that provokes the fear. This, of course, is not the case in deprivation neurosis. Here the fear is not determined by the nature of a certain object, but by the uneasiness and discomfort of the subject who feels inadequate and unable to cope with the circumstances of his life.

The fact that they cannot successfully face life and all its challenges makes them fearful. It is typical for these neurotics, and we have observed them repeatedly, that they show signs of *disintegration* whenever the *circumstances in which they live change;* for example, when they are placed in a new job, when they move to another home or town, when they live in a rooming house or apartment and get a new landlord. Having been accustomed to the old job, home, or landlord, they had acquired a certain feeling of security which they now lose as the situation changes. The new situation overwhelms them and it becomes impossible for them to go on. The same is often true for the deprivation neurotic woman when she enters into marriage, becomes pregnant, or has a baby, especially the first one.

This is not so in the case of patients with a repressive neurosis. A scrupulous person does not become more or less scrupulous on having his job assignment changed or when he moves to another neighborhood. Their fear, as such, is not determined by the circumstances, although it may be aggravated by increased demands on their time and energy due to which they have less or no time for recreation and relaxation. The fear of deprivation neurotics, however, has its root precisely in their failure to adjust to the circumstances. Therefore, from an objective point of view, the fear of deprivation neurotics is not an irrational one, for they are indeed faced with an insurmountable task.

This also explains why the fear of deprivation neurotics is not always consistent as far as its objects are concerned. That depends entirely on the circumstances in which the deprivation neurotic finds himself. The fear of repressive neurotics, on the other hand, always adds new objects, as the first repressive action expands through both *association* and *reasoning*. The consistent manner of development of this fear becomes always evident in the course of treatment. However, there is nothing resembling this in deprivation neurotics.

These, we believe, are the main psychic features of the emotional life in deprivation neurotics. And even though each actual case will, of course, manifest its own particular characteristics, the main features, which in our opinion justify the recognition of deprivation neurosis as a *clinical entity* distinct from all other neuroses, can always be detected.

*Summarizing* again the chief characteristics of deprivation neurosis, we see on the one hand: (1) an insufficiently developed emotional life, with a consequent inability to direct oneself in a normal fashion to others; (2) a feeling of uncertainty which manifests itself usually in fear; and (3) feelings of inferiority and inadequacy, with or without feelings of guilt, which lead either to depression or to aggressive behavior. On the other hand, as distinct from the repressive neuroses, we see the absence of excessive fear or energy; an open, uninhibited attitude toward sense goods; and a static clinical symptomatology.

1—Readers not familiar with the original edition or *The Neurosis in the Light of Rational Psychology* by Terruwe, translated by Baars (Kenedy, N.Y., 1960) are advised that we do not agree with Freud that the super-ego constitutes the repressing factor in neurosis. Repression in neurosis occurs when one of the emotions, most often, though not exclusively, fear or energy (our term for the emotions of courage and hope) interferes with and prevents other emotions from running their natural course. This course is essentially one of wanting to be guided by reason and will. It is precisely this process with which fear and/or energy interfere and which constitutes the fundamental neurotic repressive process.

2—*"une avidité affective," "une gloutonnerie sentimentale."*

# CHAPTER IV

# SENSE IMPAIRMENTS, LACK OF ORDER, FATIGUE

In addition to symptoms pertaining to the emotional life of deprivation neurotic patients, there are also certain characteristic deviations in their sensory cognitive life as well as in their external conduct.

The function of the sensory cognitive powers, the external and internal senses, is influenced strongly by the emotional life. At least this appears to be the case. Physically the organs and senses of these patients grow in a normal manner, and their potential functioning equals that of normal persons. Yet the actual functioning may be strongly hampered by the retarded emotional life. Whether and to what extent this occurs will depend, of course, entirely on the person's constitution and on the circumstances in which he lives.

First we will consider the most primitive of the external senses: touch, taste, and smell. Then the higher senses of vision and hearing will be discussed.

## SENSE OF TOUCH

The tactile sense in deprivation neurotic patients usually has not been sufficiently developed as a result of inadequate tactile tenderness by the mother. This may manifest itself in different ways. One of our female patients, for example, had a completely undeveloped sense of touch. At a certain stage in her therapy she began to experience the touch of a soft object as pleasing to her, following which she got an urge to touch everything in her surroundings. Another girl, a student, once wrote us: "I always have to touch somebody, to feel him. I am even inclined to do it with my teachers, but I always forget that this is not the proper thing to do. But once I have touched you, I become calm and happy. Sometimes I need that so badly."

One may see *strange things* in this respect. One of our patients, a young man twenty years old, was hardly able to let go of things which he touched. Objects, in a manner of speaking, took hold of him. It took him hours to dress because he kept holding on to each piece of clothing. When he wanted to put away a book, he could not get rid of it. In his work as an electrician this peculiar phenomenon was not without danger, but fortunately his compulsion to grip objects was less intense when somebody was around or observing him. In our opinion, this symptom was the manifestation of his need for some form of contact, and this contact was realized by holding on to an object compulsively. In the presence of another person, the compulsion lost some of its intensity through the diversion caused by interpersonal contact.

A similar symptom was seen in another patient who had the greatest difficulty in disposing of cigarette butts. Prior to therapy for his deprivation neurosis, when his sense of touch was still completely undeveloped, he had been able to throw away his cigarette butts without any trouble. But when the tactile sense began to grow, he no longer could let go of them; he was so intimately connected with his cigarettes, because he had held them in his mouth, that in a certain sense it was a traumatic experience to be separated from them. And each time he lit a cigarette he dreaded the moment when he would have to dispose of what was left of it.

One of the case histories further on in this book describes a man who had such difficulty in letting go of playing cards that each time he shuffled the cards he had a hard time stopping.

### SENSE OF TASTE

The sense of taste is closely associated with the tactile sense.

Here also one may see a total nondevelopment in serious cases of deprivation neurosis. Such people swallow their food without being aware of its taste. In therapy, when the sense of taste begins to develop, these patients frequently get an intense urge to eat *sweets*. Of course, it is well known that this urge often represents a manifestation of a frustrated sexual drive, but this is not the case for these patients. Interestingly enough, they first develop an unmistakable preference for the kind of sweets that children like best, the sticky variety. Bonbons and such have little appeal. It is well known that the sense of taste is based on that of touch, and in these patients one could almost say that their enjoyment of sweets derives even more from the stimulation of the tactile than of the gustatory sense. The following letter from the aforementioned girl student illustrates this very clearly.

> Doctor, I have been thinking some more about my desire for sweets. What kind do I like best? Licorice, caramels, and chewy gingerbread. And when do I crave them most? When I feel lonesome, when I have a need to be with someone. Those feelings may come all of a sudden. You suddenly want to be close to somebody, but there is no one. Of course, you are not always conscious of these needs; it is some vague kind of feeling of wanting to reach out for someone or something, and it is in those moments that you reach for the candy. And the more you have in your mouth, the better it is; in fact, you have to force yourself to stop, for otherwise you would eat everything at once until there would be nothing left.
>
> I wonder whether one unconsciously gropes for the sense of taste when the tactile sense is not being satisfied. After all, babies want to suck or eat all the time. Licorice and caramels all have a sticky, chewy quality which prolongs the pleasant sensation in your mouth. The contact with these substances is really intense, and the more you have in your mouth the more intense is this contact. I

believe that actually the chewing provides more joy than the taste.

Another patient told us that at first her greatest desire was for children's candy, and always in large quantities: a full mouth of taffy, licorice, jujubes, English toffees, sugar cookies, and cotton candy.

### SENSE OF SMELL

At times the sense of smell may also be the subject of peculiar manifestations. One of our female patients wrote us about her experiences: "When I receive a letter from you, the first thing I do is to smell it for fifteen minutes or so that I may feel your presence by smelling your soap. And when what you have written me is also good, I am really happy, so happy that I start sniffing at all the things in my room just like a little dog. At that time, there is nothing I'd rather do for an hour or an hour and a half." When the same patient receives a letter from the clergyman who helps her a great deal, she sniffs at it to see what kind of cigars or cigarettes he was smoking at the time of writing.

And this is what another girl wrote about this subject: "Already a long time has elapsed since I used to sniff everything. My mother (the lady who had taken it upon herself to care for her as a mother) even called me her 'little dog.' I liked to sniff her and her special scent made me feel good. It was more than just the desire for being coddled and protected. And when I was with you, I did not merely seek to be safe and secure, but also I looked for the familiar pleasant scent which I had observed in the few letters you were so kind to send me. The printed cards I got from you have very little of this scent, as your hands did not touch them long enough."

### SENSE OF SIGHT

At times the sensations from these three lower senses determine the impression the patient receives of another person. For example, one patient could never remember what we looked like or which dress we had worn. She was well aware of the touch of our hand when we had shaken hands. She also retained the feeling of our dress or coat or chair when she had touched them. The smell of the soap used on our hands was vivid to her, but she simply could not recall our face. We have made similar observations in quite a few patients. Because they only retain tactile sense impressions, they sometimes ask us for a photograph so that they may know what we look like when we are not with them. Cases like these show clearly that the so-called lower senses are the first to develop fully. As far as the visual sense is concerned in these cases, only visual perception is adequate, while visual engram formation is apparently impaired and the function of ekphorizing or recalling the visual engrams is altogether lacking.[1] Thus, while the lower senses possess these three functions in their entirety, the sense of vision has to develop them as yet.

Another interesting case of impaired visual sense was that of a woman teacher who had been away from her city of residence for a few years and upon her return did not recognize its huge cathedral, although in the past she had visited it hundreds of times.

As far as the sense of hearing is concerned, no special observations have been made.

### DIFFUSE OBSERVATION

We have also noticed that deprivation neurotics often observe what they see only diffusely. For instance, it may take several years before they notice an antique cupboard in our consultation room, a picture on the wall, or a brooch that one of us wears regularly. Once, when a new carpet had been laid in our consultation room, several patients remarked, "Doctor, what has happened here? It seems as if something is different, but I don't know what." None of them was able to say exactly what change had taken place! Often such patients ask such questions as, "Was this painting always here?" or "Has this carpet always been orange?"

Obsessive-compulsive neurotics, on the other hand, see and observe things very accurately, especially defects, as for example a chip in an ashtray, a streak on the wall of a freshly painted room, a picture that doesn't hang straight.

Werner[2] describes how children observe in a diffuse manner; they see the whole without the details. If this is true for all children, it would be another confirmation of the retarded development of deprivation neurotic patients.

INTERNAL SENSES

As far as the internal senses are concerned, we have observed frequent impairment in deprivation neurotics of the ability to form engrams. These disturbances of "impressibility" vary in intensity at different periods during their illness. One very intelligent patient had experienced much difficulty during his high school studies. While he had done well in mathematics and somewhat less so in languages, he had never been able to get passing marks in history and geography. It is precisely in these subjects that *engram formation and memory* are extremely important. But the remarkable thing was that when he recovered from his deprivation neurosis, he proved to have an excellent memory for concrete facts!

A girl who had never known her mother, and who since infancy had been brought up in an orphanage, appeared to have learned little or nothing in grade school. Although of considerable innate intelligence she was unable to learn anything, but when her deprivation neurosis improved considerably in therapy, she was able to make up for lost time.

A most unusual case was that of two sisters. The older girl had received much affection from her mother and was always at the top of her class. Her much younger sister, however, had been only several weeks old when the father was arrested by the Nazis and executed for his work in the Dutch underground.

This terrible fate had affected the mother of the girls to such a degree that she developed a severe and long-lasting depression during which she neglected her home and children. As a result, the younger girl had been deprived of all motherly affection and tender care, and she developed a most severe deprivation neurosis. In spite of the fact that psychological testing had shown her to be of above-average intelligence, she was always one of the poorest students in her class. She simply could not learn.[3]

On a few occasions we noticed that a patient possessed a good or even excellent intellectual engram formation, i.e., an engram formation based on ideas and abstract thoughts. At the same time, his purely sensory, mechanical engram formation of such concrete facts as telephone numbers, automobile license numbers, and multiplication tables, was also good or superior. Yet, he had the greatest difficulty in associating some abstract thought with something concrete. For instance, when he had to apply a general rule which he understood well to certain concrete facts, he would not remember which facts fell under the general rule and which constituted an exception to the rule. This disturbance is typical for such patients because in them the sensitive life has *failed to adapt to and become integrated* with the intellectual life.

A good example of such a disturbance was that of a lawyer who found it nearly impossible in his practice to apply abstract ideas to concrete facts. In making up a contract of sale of some acreage, he was unable to apply the rules governing such a contract to the facts given to him by his client. Even the distinction between the concept of creditor and debtor, when it had to be applied to a concrete case, created so much confusion that he was unable to draw up the necessary legal papers. As a result of this man's arrested emotional development, his concrete sense knowledge had not been integrated with his abstract universal knowledge. Both could be said to operate independently of each other without the normal subordination of sense knowledge to universal knowledge.

Another patient showed this disturbance in a different area.

He was unable to recall the feelings of others, not even those of his fiancee. When they had been out together, he had not the slightest recollection of the feelings she had expressed during the evening!

In other cases there is not the slightest sign of a disturbance of engram formation. In fact, it may be considered excellent. Or, as happens occasionally, engram formation may be good but only for a certain period. This occurred in a very able nurseryman who had quit his work for several years and then discovered that he had forgotten everything he ever knew about it. And a teacher who had not been actively engaged in her profession for a number of years had to learn everything anew before she was able to return to the classroom.

These are the deviations that we have observed in the cognitive life of deprivation neurotics. What about their external behavior? Here, too, we have seen some characteristic manifestations.

LACK OF ORDER

One such manifestation is the fact that they often are surrounded by hopeless disorder. In one of our patients, a student at the university, this lack of order was so pronounced that it was well known among all his fellow students. Another patient, a young girl, was given a room of her own by members of her family so that she could make as much of a mess as she wanted. When sharing a room with someone else she was totally unable to give any semblance of neatness to her part of the room. Again, another patient wrote the following letter to us:

> Doctor, my room is simply chaos; it looks worse every day. I constantly mean to clean it up a little, but that is as far as I get. This morning my umbrella was on the table and I thought, "The Doctor should see this!" Since I have been living alone it has become steadily worse. When I get up in the morning I don't know what I should do first; and now that I have to fix my own meals and do the

dishes too, I am completely at a loss. I just stack the dirty dishes from one day to the next until there is no room left in the kitchen. I know that I should wash them but it never gets done. Right now I have no idea where to put things any more and just sit around to get some rest from all the thinking I do about it. I would like to have a good cry about it; I know that would help, but I can't do it at the moment. Sometimes I force myself to fix things a little bit even to the point of getting out of breath, but all that it amounts to is a rearrangement of the mess for I just don't know where I should put things.

Doctor, it is really true but I loathe going to bed at night, for my bed looks like a bundle of rags. When I lie in bed surrounded by hot water bottles, I think, 'The first thing I'll do in the morning is to make my bed,' for it is such a mess that I can't even straighten out the blankets. But when I open my eyes in the morning and see the mess my bed is in, I despair of ever straightening it out and leave it at that.

At first when female patients complained during their interviews that their houses were always in disorder and their closets stacked so full that every time they opened the door things would tumble down, while their husbands could not find their ties or socks in the drawers in the bedroom, we were not inclined to take these complaints very seriously, especially as these women usually impressed us as personally neat rather than untidy. We tried to reassure them that things probably were not as bad as they thought until we began to hear from various husbands that the chaos at their home was indeed indescribable.

In many cases the husbands' stories even exceeded those of the women. One husband of a deprivation neurotic patient took pictures of every room in the house, including the basement. Nothing was in place, no bed was made up, drawers were open, clothing was strewn haphazardly over the living room floor and furniture, toys, and books and magazines littered the stairs, there was no chair, sofa, or bed which one could have occupied without first removing boxes, shoes, appliances, cans, or dishes. Luggage used for a trip six months before was still lying around open and half full.

The patient, a very intelligent and talented woman, whose children have not had a friend over to their house for years, wrote: "Doctor, can you imagine those poor, dear children having no discipline? They have no rules to follow as I really do not care deeply enough, emotionally, to carry any rules through. I have made rules many times, posted them on walls to help the children remember, but I forget to enforce anything. I have spent my entire life thinking, instead of doing . . . This place is so junky, it is hard to walk in without falling over something. It is almost too much effort to hang up my coat, but I do manage that at least (the children don't). We are walking on piles of dirty clothes, clean clothes, toys, books, all over, everywhere. When the children ask for clothes I just drag them out of a pile somewhere."

It is from such cases that we began to realize how well this manifestation fits into the deprivation neurosis syndrome. *To bring order into things* is a matter of arranging concrete things according to a plan, of the intellectual order dealing with the sensory order. But it is just this, the penetration of the sensory order by the intellectual order, which is lacking in deprivation neurotics.

Sometimes these patients have some sort of principle to guide them in arranging things, but instead of creating order, this principle will do exactly the opposite. For instance, in preparing a meal, they have everything close at hand so all they need to do is reach. But for someone who is used to an orderly system, their arrangement of things appears as haphazard and cluttered.

Not only do these patients frequently fail to have order around them, they also find it extremely difficult to direct their actions toward an orderly whole. To write examination papers and to go through all the points of a program are some examples. One patient was the secretary of several societies and as such had to keep the minutes of each meeting. During his interviews he always complained that he could not work out these minutes for the next meeting. Another patient suddenly became confused and fearful after he conceived the idea of writing a little book about a subject which he had mastered completely. He never finished writing it. In all these cases the difficulty is the same in essence: intellectually the patients have to *bring order into material things*, and that is something for which they are not yet prepared.

Finally, it must be mentioned that some patients with extremely severe deprivation neuroses experience a great reluctance to start practicing the profession for which they have been trained, despite acquired titles and other proofs of professional qualifications. They just cannot make themselves assume the responsibility, presumably because of a deep inner feeling of being unfit and not really up to the demands of their work.

### PHYSICAL STATUS

The strictly physical life of patients with deprivation neuroses also deserves a few words, if only to state that we have found few, if any, characteristic peculiarities. Their appearance is generally *more youthful* than their chronological age would indicate. In several cases the nailbeds of these patients seemed to have retained a childish stage of development.

We are also of the opinion that the *tics* which occur so frequently in repressive neuroses do not belong to the syndrome of the deprivation neurosis. When they do occur, they must be considered symptomatic of a superimposed pseudoneurotic reaction, or, in other words, the result of circumstances to which the patient has difficulty adapting himself. One of our patients, for example, complained that she began to exhibit certain tics during our vacation periods, which always were times of considerable difficulty for her. But as soon as she learned that we had returned from our vacation, for instance, when she passed our house in the evening and saw the lights burning there, the tics disappeared immediately.

A subjective feeling of *fatigue* is a frequent observation in these patients. In many it grows into a state of utter exhaustion for which they consult their physician. If any organic reasons for fatigue are discovered—anemia, hypothyroidism, relative hypoglycemia, and so forth—these are usually incidental since corrective treatment only partially alleviates the fatigue. The main cause of such fatigue is psychological. Finding little enjoyment in life, little repose and relaxation in the joy of friendship and love, the energy of such patients is directed at achievement to counteract their deep feelings of inferiority, at pleasing others to gain their love and approval. As they readily exaggerate these energetic pursuits it is not surprising that they feel continually fatigued. If the more fearful deprivation neurotics attempt to spend the little energy they have in similar ways, they seem to complain less of fatigue, perhaps because they have never known the protracted periods of high energy of the more energetic patients, and thus take their lifelong low fatigue threshold for granted.

A typical example of the former was a farmer in his mid-twenties who sought help because of extreme fatigue which made it necessary to quit his work altogether, this in spite of an excellent physique, a strong, muscular build, and a history of having done heavy labor without discomfort since early childhood. Exhaustive laboratory and other studies failed to find an organic cause for his fatigue, which gradually got worse even when he found employment in which he was not required to do strenuous physical work.

The *sleep* of deprivation neurotics is usually not disturbed; they have no difficulty falling asleep and sleep soundly all night long unless a repressive neurosis or a pseudoneurotic reaction has been superimposed on the deprivation neurosis. This may be a helpful clue in the differential diagnosis of fear neurosis, for sleep disturbances are a frequent phenomenon in the latter. The dream life of deprivation neurotics seems to lack any special features which would distinguish it from other types of neuroses.

1—See also Eugen P. Blueler, *Textbook of Psychiatry* (New York: Dover Publications, 1951), pp. 28-29: "Everything that has been physically experienced leaves behind a lasting trace, or engram. We recognize this by the fact that the more often a process has been repeated the easier it runs off . . . and above all that one remembers psychic processes. What modification the engram represents we do not know. In remembering something there must be a recurrence of a function resembling a previous experience . . . like the repetition of a practiced motion. We designate this as an ekphoria of the engrams . . . The ability to form engrams, the engraphia, was designated by Sernicke as 'impressibility' (*merkfähig-keit*) . . . and this has been hazily contrasted with 'memory.' Memory in this connection no longer means the whole memory . . . but the . . . ability to ekphorize the engrams."

2—*Op. cit.* p. 87.

3—It is possible that learning difficulties in intelligent children are not infrequently based on a deprivation neurosis. It might be worthwhile for school psychologists to investigate this further.

# CHAPTER V

# DON'T LET THE PSYCHIATRIST TELL YOU THAT YOU ARE SCHIZOPHRENIC, IF YOU ARE ONLY A DEPRIVATION NEUROTIC

It may happen in certain cases that some of the clinical symptoms of deprivation neurosis manifest themselves in such a pronounced manner that the initial impression given is that of a different clinical syndrome.

## PARANOID CONDITION

For example, several of our patients seemed to suffer from a paranoid condition (sensitive paranoia of Kretschmer). Chapter VIII contains an extensive case history of a deprivation neurotic priest who felt that people were plotting against him, suspected newspaper articles of making references to him, and believed that there were hidden recording devices in the doctor's examination room. We refer the reader to this case report for a more detailed discussion of the differential diagnostic aspects.

Another case, also at first resembling a paranoid condition, was that of a young man who came to us because of excessive masturbation. He lived over a local bar in a small town, and had come to think that the barkeeper had found out about his masturbation and was telling all his customers about it. Finally, he had gotten the idea that the whole town knew about it and was talking about him behind his back.

A similar case, which also proved to be a deprivation neurosis on further examination, was that of a woman who thought that instruments had been installed in her car so that someone could hear and see everything she said and did. Out of fear she tried to convince this alleged spy that she had nothing to hide by mentioning aloud the names of all the towns and villages through which she drove on her various trips. Whenever she noticed people with much make-up or unusual wearing apparel around her, she also experienced the delusion that someone was making a movie of her life, and that these people were actors in the movie.

Still another woman, a clear-cut deprivation neurotic, was firmly convinced that she had strange-looking eyes, and that the whole town considered her appearance a disgrace. Yet in our office she was always calm, and we did not find out about these delusional ideas until one day our dog happened to bark when she came in, and she said, "Even your dog thinks I look terrible!" Our subsequent inquiry about the meaning of this remark revealed the presence of the aforementioned delusions.

### SCHIZOPHRENIC REACTIONS

Other deprivation neurotics make a schizophrenic impression, particularly when they are in a state of *confusion* or *disintegration*. Under unfavorable circumstances the basic feeling of insecurity with which they live may become intensified, and then it leads to a confusional state which resembles schizophrenia. Such a case presented itself when a young woman came to us who had been diagnosed as schizophrenic by two experienced psychiatrists. We recognized her case as a typical deprivation neurosis, treated her accordingly, and she recovered completely in time. Her subsequent marriage was a happy one, and the poise and ease with which she moved in social circles contributed greatly to the success of her husband's work. She withstood successfully, without a recurrence of her neurosis, even serious difficulties that developed as a result of circumstances beyond her control.

A thirty-year-old woman, whom we treated for deprivation neurosis, got along reasonably well in general except for periods of excessive masturbation. These repeated acts made her extremely fearful, as is typical of many patients with this type of neurosis. Whenever they do something that is objectively wrong, for which subjectively they are not to blame, they develop intense feelings of guilt and concomitant pathological fears. In one of these periods her intense fears made her so confused that her relatives became concerned and had her taken to a psychiatric hospital, but without notifying us. Later, when we were informed of this development, her physician told us that she had been admitted as schizophrenic, but that he had come to doubt this diagnosis gradually because of her good emotional rapport.

An internationally known psychiatrist referred a young man to us for treatment of "an early schizophrenic breakdown, as he was tense, withdrawn, vague, preoccupied, and had spent the greater part of each day 'just thinking,' yet there was no evidence of thought disorganization, delusions, or hallucinations." One of the psychological tests taken by the patient was reported by a member of the psychiatrist's staff as follows: "This individual displays a strong need to portray himself in a favorable light. He may be expected to be evasive and/or uncooperative. The profile is psychotic rather than neurotic, although he has considerable anxiety which he is struggling to cope with by his obsessive-compulsive defenses. There is presently no evidence of thought disorganization. Similar profiles among our patients have been diagnosed schizophrenic."

The young man proved to be a typical deprivation neurotic, although he also had a superimposed obsessive-compulsive neurosis. He responded well to therapy, became a successful teacher, and at last report was happily married with two children.

In this connection it is important to mention the book *Symbolic Realization*,[1] in which M. A. Sechehaye describes the case of a schizophrenic girl whom she treated in a special manner. She simultaneously showed the girl motherly love and symbolically fulfilled the patient's wishes. As a result of this manner of treatment, the girl recovered completely. We must ask the question: Wasn't it more likely that this girl was a deprivation neurotic rather than a schizophrenic?

### HYSTERICAL NEUROSIS

The hysterical neurosis is the third diagnostic category which the clinician will at times consider when first confronted with a deprivation neurotic, especially in cases in which the patient's need for attention assumes an unusually conspicuous form.

An excellent example of such a case was an intelligent, but formally uneducated twenty-four-year-old young woman, referred to us by her family physician because she tried to gain attention by artificial means. She possessed an immense urge to express herself, but was able to realize this urge only in her physical appearance. Her first appointment with us was at eight o'clock in the morning, and in spite of a pouring rain and the early hour, she appeared in a flowing cocktail dress and elaborate make-up. She had been diagnosed as a hysterical psychopath in a psychiatric clinic elsewhere, but her muscle stretch reflexes were such that this diagnosis seemed highly unlikely. The family physician, who had known the girl for many years, had not been in favor of this diagnosis, and although he too had been impressed by her intense urge to express herself, his feelings had rebelled against the label of "hysterical show-off." Our examination soon made it evident that we were dealing with a deprivation neurotic girl who had been denied every token of love by her mother. The latter, by the way, was seen at a later date and strongly impressed us with being a deprivation neurotic herself. In this case there was no hysterical psychopathic basis for the girl's need to draw attention to herself; this was merely an exaggerated form of the desire that others would direct themselves to her.

Certain people with little formal education often convert their expressive needs in *somatic symptoms*. Through learning, matter is so kneaded that it becomes a fit vehicle for the expression of man's aspirations, which are always more or less spiritual. But without education and the learning process, matter is not offered this possibility. No option is left but to use matter itself for one's expressive needs. This then may well take the form of conversion reactions.

So it was in the case of this girl. The attention she sought was an attention to which she was in a certain sense entitled, for she needed it for the natural development of her emotional life.

Although such people have a need for contact with others, they are not able to form contacts in a normal manner. Consequently they seek attention from those who by virtue of their vocation direct themselves to others—usually the clergyman and the physician. These patients frequently go from one doctor to the other and from one cleric to the next. Such behavior is usually considered hysterical, but in deprivation neurotics this is certainly not true.

### PERSONALITY DISORDERS

A fourth distinction to be made, often with considerable difficulty, is that of the maladaptive pattern of living which characterizes the personality disorders. We have in mind particularly the sub-types of the hysterical personality, paranoid personality and the pathological liar. The hysterical personality manifests behavior which closely resembles that of the hysterical neurotic and some deprivation neurotics. The differential diagnosis cannot be made on the basis of their respective superficial clinical behavioral manifestation, but depends on the recognition of the fundamental characteristics of the person with a personality disorder; a life-long pattern of extreme selfishness, impulsiveness, marked emotional liability and a seeming inability to learn from experience. Knowledge of this basic symptomatology is also essential for differentiating the paranoid personality from a paranoid psychosis or a deprivation neurosis with paranoid behavior.

Perhaps the most difficult differential diagnosis of all is that between the pathological liar—one particular type of psychopathic personality[2] and the unaffirmed person who utilizes his superior intellect and talents for the purpose of affirming himself by means of power and fame—if not also by any of the other means described in *Born Only Once*.[3]

The pathological liar is the type of person who imagines and tells the most fantastic stories, thereby leading others to believe in things which have no counterpart in reality. Although the stories of all psychopathic personalities are untrustworthy, due to the fact that man's imagination is strongly influenced by the emotions which in their case however are not penetrated and governed by reason, in the pathological liar or *pseudologia phantastica* it is clinically the most outstanding feature. His creative imagination is so susceptible to stimulation that, without any effort at all, he is able to invent and tell complicated and fictitious stories which impress almost everybody as being true. History has recorded several famous or notorious, but always colorful impostors and swindlers like "Count" Cagliostro, while others make the headlines from time to time in our present age when exposed as individuals who, for example, posed alternately as a high ranking military officer, physician, government expert and so on until by chance exposed.

We are acquainted with several unaffirmed persons whose attempts to convince others, and perhaps also themselves, of their significance and self-worth have resulted in behavior reminiscent of that of the pathological liar. One of the most interesting cases was that of a young unaffirmed priest of humble origin who had everyone, including his superiors, believe that he was the most trustworthy, sincere, dedicated and prayerful person even when telling lies, pursuing his selfish interests and neglecting his duties. Because of his success in the latter he had alienated most of his peers as they were left doing the pastoral work he shunned in his feverish accumulation of academic degrees. These he displayed everywhere in an ostentatious manner in his futile attempts at self-affirmation. The few clients he counseled, all selected carefully according to his personal preferences and rather inept counseling ability, would sooner or later feel betrayed by his pseudo-affirming attitude aimed at gaining their affection and admiration.

He was able to control many of his co-workers by intimidation and manipulation, and by using against them the information he obtained by listening behind doors during their counseling sessions, or by steaming open their mail, or listening in on their telephone conversations. By manipulating accounts and defrauding others he was able to live in grand style, surrounded by status symbols and having his breakfast served in bed by the housekeeper. Some of his more intelligent, but probably emotionally deprived or unstable co-workers who were consciously aware of his lust for power and control over others, themselves included, were unable or afraid to resist or expose him. In the case of women co-workers he cleverly manipulated their love-hate feelings toward him, even to the point of inducing severe depressions. One of these women would tell others in her more self-possessed moments that she realized full well that "the power of his position had gone to his head," and that she "did not trust him." At times she was overheard to say after listening to one of his admittedly moving homilies at the liturgy that "she wished that he would practice what he preached." On one occasion when she had been goaded by him into a deep depression she swore that she would restrict her future contacts with him to her work as a secretary in his office. However, several months later she was seen again sharing his social life, an apparent victim of the charm he exercised over her.

In his ability to impress others with his presumed talents and power this desperately self-affirming priest rivaled the innate talent of the typical pathological liar. One of the students at the nearby seminary where he taught was absolutely convinced that he actually was a bishop. This, the priest had told him in the strictest of confidence, had come about shortly before he was to go on a university-sponsored post-graduate tour to Russia. He had been summoned to Rome where he was consecrated a bishop in secret ceremony so he would be able to ordain some Russian deacons if he were successful in evading the ubiquitous police-guides. On his return from his highly successful mission, so he had told the young seminarian, he had been received in private audience by the Pope who had embraced him with tears in his eyes and called him "his brother." As if this was not enough to impress the gullible seminarian the priest spoke occasionally of being invited by visiting bishops and cardinals for participating in their discussions on highly confidential ecclesiastical matters.

What distinguishes this unaffirmed priest with such pronounced psychopathic-like behavior from the true constitutional psychopath is the absence of the clinical triad of psychopathic symptoms: extreme selfishness, impulsivity and unpredictable, sudden mood changes. By and large this triad was absent in this priest. Another helpful diagnostic hint in this case was the observation that young people disliked him from the moment they first met him in spite of his efforts to act like a friendly and mature priest. Contrary to many adult persons these youngsters could sense the lack of authenticity of his behavior that served to mask his feelings of inferiority and inadequacy. It has been our experience that outgoing psychopathic liars and swindlers are liked by all they come in contact with. This is probably due to the fact that in them there is no discrepancy between their feelings and behavior.

1—New York: International University Press, 1951.

2—See "Psychopathic Personality and Neurosis," by Anna A. Terruwe, translated by Conrad W. Baars, M.D., T. J. Kenedy & Sons, N. Y., 1958.

3—Conrad W. Baars, M.D., Franciscan Herald Press, Chicago, Illinois. 1975.

# CHAPTER VI

# WHAT KIND OF THERAPY DO DEPRIVATION NEUROTICS NEED?

In the unabridged edition we explained that the proper therapy of the repressive neuroses, which result from repression of the pleasure emotions by the emotions of the utility appetite, must be directed at lessening the abnormal action of the repressing emotions of fear or energy. Only when this is accomplished, is it possible for the arrested emotional life to resume its growth toward maturity.

It is immediately evident that this approach cannot possibly apply to the therapy of deprivation neurosis, for in this neurosis there is no repression and thus no abnormal action by excessive fear or energy. This illness is not caused by repression, but rather by the fact that the conditions for normal development of the emotional life were lacking during childhood. Frustration of the child's essential need for loving acceptance leads to a standstill in his emotional growth which in turn produces the various clinical symptoms described elsewhere in this book. Therefore, a causal therapy of deprivation neurosis must be directed first of all at an optimal restoration of those conditions which make it possible for the emotional life to resume its natural growth. Secondly, therapy must aim at keeping this growing process in the proper channels.

Man's growth is a natural process and the same is true for the resumed growth which is the aim in the treatment of the deprivation neurotic. Whenever nature is prevented from unfolding it will resume its rightful course as soon as it is given an opportunity and the proper conditions are created. Foremost among these for the child is the *affirmation*[1] of his being. Every child is completely dependent; left to himself, he is psychologically incapable of coping with life. He needs to be accepted and protected by someone else. Not until then will he feel safe and able to deal with life. The child must feel that someone is so concerned with him that he has been drawn, so to speak, into the safety of the orbit of that someone's life. Only then is the void of the child's dependency filled, only then is he in a condition in which natural growth and development can take place.

## EMOTIONAL AFFIRMATION

In the normal and natural course of events, this condition is brought about when the child feels the love of his parents. In the earliest years, this love will mainly be that of his mother, but when the child grows older, it will also include the dedicated and loving concern of his father. As a baby, the child can experience this love, this affirmation of its being, only by way of the sense of touch, for the other senses have not yet sufficiently developed. For this reason it is very important for the child's psychic development that the mother should *caress and cuddle* the baby and in these ways make the baby feel her love. These, and all other tactile manifestations of motherly tenderness, are as necessary for the psychic growth of the child as milk is for his physical growth.

In later years the child must also be affirmed by the father. Here again the affirmation must be expressed in a tactile manner, although verbal affirmation by this time has assumed an even greater role. Generally, there is a difference between boys and girls in this respect. Tactile affirmation is of even greater importance for girls than for boys, although the latter cannot do without it. Perhaps this is due to the fact that, in general, the emotional life of the man is more deeply penetrated by reason than that of the woman. This would explain why boys have a

greater need for intellectual affirmation than do girls, for whom
the tenderness of emotional affirmation plays the more important
role. No wonder then that the lack of affirmation by the father
causes greater psychological trauma in boys than in girls.

But no matter which explanation is correct, the fact remains
that both boys and girls need emotional affirmation, and that
the lack of this leads, of necessity, to the development of a
deprivation neurosis. When persons with such a neurosis seek
the help of a psychiatrist, he must first, if he is to start them on
the road to recovery, give them the emotional affirmation which
they did not receive in their childhood. In other words, he must
make them experience the feelings of affection which others did
not give them. As far as this feeling is concerned, they are still
totally dependent and incapable of dealing with life by themselves. Therefore, they must come to *feel*[2] that they are not
alone, and that there is someone to whom they can entrust
themselves, with whom they are really safe. But they develop
this feeling in regard to the therapist only when they feel in
the literal sense of the word, when they sense that he has sympathy and affection for them. The knowledge that the therapist
is an able and well-qualified person has no bearing on this; such
knowledge moves only their intellectual faculty, not their feelings. It is precisely in their feelings that they need to be affirmed.
They feel safe only when they sense that they themselves mean
something to the therapist's feelings and that he also has sympathy for them as human beings. As long as the therapist has a
business-like attitude toward such patients, his therapy will be
of no avail. In such a relationship they cannot feel safe; they
remain uncertain and, thus, incapable of growing.

The therapist must really feel sympathetic toward his patient,
and while fully respecting the therapist-patient relationship, he
must be able to show this sympathy in a manner which the
patient can feel. The therapist must express this affection through
cordiality, personal interest and concern, dedication, patience;
in short, in every way in which a father and a mother show
love for their child. Patients really feel toward their therapist

the way a child does toward his parent. The therapist's affection, which must be demonstrated without any violation of the professional relationship, is a matter of the utmost significance for the patient and a subject about which he is extremely sensitive. The patient is aware of the fact that it is the therapist's affection for him which he needs most of all. Because of this he views everything that the therapist says and does as evidence as to whether or not the therapist loves him. Every shortcoming on the part of the therapist in this regard, even the slightest and most unintentional one, may be interpreted by the patient as proof that the therapist does not care for him, that he is merely a number as far as the therapist is concerned. Such reactions, of course, always create the greatest difficulties and conflicts, and demand the utmost patience and tact from the therapist. Some patients even test the therapist in a more or less systematic fashion to see whether he really cares for them!

### INTELLECTUAL AFFIRMATION

Although the emotional affirmation of the patient afforded by the therapist's feelings of sympathy is the primary requirement in the recovery process, it is not sufficient for the adult patient. Such affirmation by the mother's tender love is sufficient for a baby because the baby's life needs are still very limited. In the adult, the life of the intellect, of awareness and introspection, has grown uninterruptedly, and the uncertainty which first developed in his emotional life has extended itself to all other aspects of his life. For this reason, the deprivation neurotic patient requires more than the therapist's affection; he has to be affirmed in every aspect of his life and must come to feel that he does not stand alone in all matters. Consequently, he will have a need to *obtain approval* by telling the therapist about everything in his life about which he is uncertain. One of our patients, a teacher, wrote down everything he did during the week in a little notebook. At every visit he would recount all the events which occurred since his previous treatment so that we could approve everything. An even more striking example of this need concerned the patient whose case history is the second given in Chapter VIII of this book. Not only did we have to affirm all her activities, but she would not rest until she had shown us everything she had worn and used, and we had given our approval.

These patients have an even stronger need to be affirmed as far as their own persons are concerned. It is necessary to destroy the reasons which make them consider themselves bad. They must learn that nothing can damage the therapist's favorable opinion of them or his affection for them. Little by little they must tell the therapist everything about their lives, about all the things which they feel make them bad and inferior. This is also necessary in treating repressive neuroses, but for another reason: namely, to obtain a *discharge* or *abreaction* for their emotions. In deprivation neurosis, however, patients need to know not only that the therapist knows them through and through, even in regard to what they consider their worst qualities, but also that, in spite of this knowledge, he retains his affection for them. It is only as a result of this experience that these patients will feel affirmed in everything. As long as there remains some area in which this has not taken place, they will not be able to accept completely the therapist's opinion of themselves, and that, after all, is the goal of therapy. Frequently this takes a long time, because the patients are fearful of losing the therapist's affection, and they *hide themselves* from him in regard to whatever causes them the greatest conflicts and worries. But when their confidence increases gradually, all these things will come to the fore and will be told to the therapist.

Obviously, the therapist must avoid being aggressive in this respect. Every attempt to probe and to urge patients to reveal themselves frightens them, for they are extremely sensitive in such matters. The therapist must wait until the patients feel a need to unburden themselves. What we have said about this in regard to repressive neurotics pertains even more to deprivation neurotics.

## COMPARISON WITH PSYCHOANALYSIS

A systematic analytic approach should never be attempted in these cases: first, because these patients have no conflicts as such which need to be resolved, and second, because they are not at all ready for such an analysis. Fortunately, the psychologist Germaine Geux, in her aforementioned book, *La névrose d'abandon*, has also strongly emphasized this fact. She warns that these patients have not yet developed sufficiently to reach the Oedipal phase and for that reason are not susceptible to a classical analysis. Although Geux puts the idea in different terminology, her work has the great merit that it is a serious warning from the psychoanalytic side to abstain from classical psychoanalytic methods in the treatment of these patients.

The two previously explained points, emotional affirmation of the patient by the therapist's affection, and repeated and consistent intellectual affirmation by the therapist's understanding, constitute the basis for the psychic development of the patient. If he is to be cured, he must make up for what he has not yet experienced emotionally and he must do this in the gradual manner which is characteristic of the natural growth process. He must pass through all the phases of emotional development which follow up the stage at which this process was arrested as a result of frustration of his natural needs. It need hardly be stated that when this does happen, all kinds of feelings will become manifest which are foreign to the emotional life of the normal adult. It then is up to the therapist to show the patient that these newly arisen feelings are not at all strange or inferior, but that it is entirely proper and necessary for him to experience them. Every case, of course, will have its own characteristic development depending upon temperament and other constitutional factors, as well as on the external circumstances, yet the principle is the same for all.

## ENVIRONMENTAL INFLUENCES

The ultimate success of the therapy depends to a large extent on external circumstances. When these are unfavorable and the patient cannot receive what the development of his emotional life requires, the prognosis must be considered poor. For example, in the case of a patient who was deprived of motherly tenderness as a child and thus has a special need for it, everything depends on whether there is somebody who can and will give him this motherly tenderness. The same is true when the patient requires affirmation by the father. Should the patient feel the need *to play* the way a child does, the circumstances should be such that this becomes possible. Unlike the case with repressive neuroses, therefore, cures depend not only on intrapsychic processes which proceed from the therapist, but also to a great extent on external factors which are not under the therapist's control. This fact must be always kept in mind for prognostic evaluation and for determining whether one is acting correctly in undertaking treatment.

The fact that persons in the patient's immediate environment usually do not understand the nature of his illness presents a special handicap. In too many instances, they are not capable of developing such understanding. They know the patient as someone who, outwardly at least, appears adult, and they do not realize that underneath this external facade the situation is entirely different. No wonder, therefore, that they continue to *expect the patient to behave as an adult.* Even when the psychiatrist has tried to explain the nature of the illness to them, and tells them how important it is to demand no more of the patient than what he is capable of emotionally, such persons cannot always translate this knowledge into action which will not further aggravate the patient's condition. In many cases, parents and other members of the family, or, in the case of religious, the superior and members of the religious community, continue by their attitude and conduct to add to the patient's suffering and force him to withdraw further into himself.

The same is true when the patient begins to behave more like a mature adult and allows his emotions to influence his behavior in a more honest and assertive manner. It is then that the pseudomaturity of certain persons in his environment will be revealed by their non-acceptance of and objection to the patient's emerging attempts to live not as a self-effacing, other-pleasing non-entity, but as a unique individual worthy of respect and recognition. The unaffirmed religious woman who has lived for decades trying to please everyone else in her community to the point of developing a severe depression will need all her courage to face some of her fellow religious after she returns from a period spent in receiving affirmation therapy. For it is true and almost a matter of course that people expect a depressed person upon completion of psychiatric treatment to conduct himself as he used to. In fact, only too often is such resumption of his former other-pleasing ways considered proof of the *effectiveness of psychiatric therapy*. And this may be true indeed if we mean by effective psychiatric therapy merely the successful removal of the symptoms of a psychiatric condition like depression by means of drugs, electroshock therapy, or any other therapeutic means. But this would not be true, if we hold effective psychiatric therapy to include also curing the underlying mental and emotional state of the depressed person. To do so would require the recognition of the unaffirmed state as a dis-ease by the psychiatric profession and the environment. For sure, this definition is not acceptable or deemed necessary by those who view man in a secular-utilitarian philosophy of life. For them man is "well" as long as he is able to perform certain functions or hold a certain job useful to society. If he loses this ability as the result of a psychiatric condition then he will be considered recovered when psychiatric treatment has succeeded in removing this temporary psychiatric obstacle to his usefulness as a cog in the operations of the state or any other community of persons.

To view the underlying unaffirmed state as a disease requires the admission by the persons in the environment of their own unaffirmed state which is in equal need of affirmation. Unless this is done the environment will continue to deny the patient and affirm themselves, a situation which poses an unnecessary burden on the recovering patient. Such persons would do well to realize that they, the so-called normal persons, can learn much from what the formerly depressed person has to offer and would grow if they were to open themselves to affirmation by the patient. Therefore, the therapist could often best serve the entire community or a family by spending some time with all its members, prior to the return of the patient.

It is certainly not an easy matter to imagine the abnormal emotional state of deprivation neurotic patients. And, even when one understands it in theory, it is not always easy to use this knowledge in practice, for no matter how considerate and sympathetic relatives or friends may try to be, they cannot help but retain their customary manner, depending on the mood they are in, of reacting emotionally to the patient. And what is more, day-to-day contact in the home or religious community with such patients often makes burdensome demands on the environment and calls for an almost heroic degree of patience from others. At times, in fact, the condition may call for the temporary removal of the patient. This happened in the case of a severe deprivation neurotic wife and mother who did not move a finger in the household and by her behavior made the atmosphere at home unbearable for her husband and children. For the sake of the family, we finally had to hospitalize her for a long period of time. This is, of course, something which one tries to avoid if at all possible, but under certain circumstances it would be unreasonable not to take this step. In such cases it is important to make the patient understand the reasonableness of this measure, since this insight, once developed, may contribute to his further progress in therapy.

### FOSTER HOME

It remains a therapeutic requirement that the psychiatrist must attempt to improve the patient's environment as much as possible, and to make the patient's circumstances more favorable by explaining his condition and the nature of his illness to those with whom he has daily contact. In some cases it will be impossible to effect a cure unless the patient's milieu is radically changed. An example of such therapeutic necessity occurred in the case of a family in which the children lived under terrific pressure from their emotionally disturbed mother. The father, a most intelligent and understanding man, was able to absorb and deflect much of this pressure. After his death, however, there was nothing to offset the domineering attitude of the mother. The youngest girl had to be treated for a most severe deprivation neurosis due to her mother's complete lack of maternal tenderness and affection. As it was impossible to expect a change in the mother's condition, we insisted on the daughter leaving home. After a good foster home had been found for her, she began to grow emotionally and responded successfully to therapy.

On the other hand, things may get worse for the patient rather than better, if the foster home also fails him. It has happened more than once that the members of a foster home selected for a patient were not able to cope with him, in spite of their good intentions and their sincere desire to help a person in need. As a result the patient once more felt rejected and blamed himself for the fact that things did not turn out as hoped for, even when it was obvious that the foster family and at times the referring social agency had failed to grasp the nature and therapeutic requirements of his illness, and therefore had expected the patient to act much more like an adult than we had advised them he would be capable of. Whenever such a traumatic incident occurred with one of our patients, we were sadly reminded of the fact that habits and rules, attitudes and expectations, do not readily change on the part of individuals or agencies dedicated to the welfare of mentally or emotionally sick people. Only too infrequently does one encounter individuals who are blessed with the wisdom of *"forgiving others for being other,"* while more often than not, those who must rely temporarily on others for their psychic well-being, find that the path to their intended welfare is a narrow one indeed.

As we cannot overemphasize the danger of therapeutic failures inherent in detrimental milieu factors, we must discuss a few more obstacles on the road to recovery. Generally speaking, the presence in the environment of deprivation neurotic patients or individuals with their own neuroses, or more or less pronounced neurotic personality traits, must be considered a prognostically unfavorable factor. The closer the relationship between the patient and one or more of such neurotic individuals, the poorer the chances of his recovery. This factor must be given due consideration if the patient is a spouse, a member of a family, or a member of a religious community. The other spouse, the parents and relatives of the patient, or the superior and members of a religious group may all set a poor example for the patient, make unrealistic demands on him, oppose or ignore the therapist's advice, or in countless other ways discourage him from becoming well and thus different from themselves. As long as only the patient is seeing a psychiatrist, the other members of the family or community presume themselves to be "healthy" individuals whose behavior and manner of living should be emulated by the patient. This air of superiority and pseudotolerance on the part of the "healthy" members of the family or community often inflicts intense and needless suffering on the patient, even when they proclaim great understanding of his needs and difficulties, and of mental and emotional illness in general.

If the patient must live in a religious community, the difficulties are often accentuated and may well outweigh the positive aspects of group living. In religious communities the patient must live in close daily contact with other adults who represent the whole gamut of character and personality traits, from mature to immature; there are people who are more or less set in their ways, and are often bound to a rigid schedule of work and other duties. Due to transfers and changing assignments, the community as a whole is rarely stable. Too few members have the time and the patience to devote themselves to the needs of a neurotic member after their first enthusiastic attempts to come to his aid have worn off without showing much in the way of visible or lasting effects. With the passage of time the patient must resign himself to increasing signs of irritation on the part of other members, who must substitute for him when he is sick or visiting the therapist, who become impatient with his seeming relapse and with the expense and duration of his therapy, and who subtly undermine the patient's confidence in the therapist and augment his feelings of guilt for being a burden to the community, even with such well-intended remarks as, "Are you still going to that doctor; you look so healthy?" The stigma of having to see a psychiatrist is particularly heavy in those religious communities where the subjects have been *trained*—we use the term deliberately—to disregard their physical pains and aches, and to bear them in silence. In such a harsh atmosphere, it is not surprising that the religious expect themselves and others to "rise above their feelings," especially above those they have been led to believe are inferior and unbecoming to a religious. Under those circumstances the patient has to suffer the added tension and suspense of having to hide the *stigma* of being so weak and spineless that he must seek psychiatric help. Fortunately, this is only true for the early stages of treatment, for when patients come to realize they are not alone in their misery and find someone who truly cares for them as an individual, they no longer care what the community thinks, and want it to benefit from a more enlightened attitude toward emotional illness.

Some of the worst obstacles in the therapeutic process are sudden enforced interruptions or terminations of treatment by patients who are financially dependent on others. Sometimes parents withdraw their financial support because they do not approve of the change in behavior or attitude of their son or daughter, or because they cannot tolerate the patient's emerging self-confidence and consider his assertiveness a personal insult and indictment of their upbringing. Or a spouse discovers that the patient is no longer the same person he married and blames the therapist for having effected a change for the worse. Or a religious superior, without giving any reason and expecting blind obedience, suddenly forbids a subject to continue therapy.

Whereas the therapist in the first case may be able to reassure the parents of the temporary nature of the behavioral changes, or, in the second case, help the spouse to adjust to the "new" personality of his beloved, the situation is frequently more complex and difficult in the case of the religious superior. One rather extreme example was the sudden notification of one of the authors—by a superior who had always shown great compassion for and sincere interest in her subjects' emotional sufferings and need for competent help—that his professional services would no longer be needed and that all subjects already in therapy would be instructed to seek therapy elsewhere. No reason was given either then, or several months later when the subjects were suddenly given permission to resume therapy. We can only speculate that a certain political faction within the community had chosen this means of asserting its power, thereby sacrificing, wittingly or unwittingly, the well-being of fellow-religious to the furtherance of its own goals. Be this as it may, the real issue here is the needless aggravation of a patient's suffering as a direct consequence of being forced to discontinue therapy without an absolutely adequate reason. We can think of no better way to illustrate the intensity of the resulting agony than to present some excerpts from the letters written by the religious subjects involved. We do this in the sincere hope that others will be spared similar suffering in the future.

> Doctor, I still can't believe it all really happened. I feel so hurt. I'm sorry for not writing sooner. I guess I was too stunned to do anything, but you have been in my daily thoughts and prayers. I could write a book about all that has happened since you were taken away from me. It would be called "Waiting"—waiting for the day when all this agony and suffering will be unmasked so that my joy may shine through . . . By the time I got to see my superior I had already suffered so much inside that I hardly knew what I was doing or saying. I still don't know why it happened. It will be most difficult to ever return to the

motherhouse because it pains me to think of having to go near the place. What an injustice—to allow human beings to continue to suffer so that WORK and EDUCATION can triumph while its members remain useful! The only thing the superior said was that she had been reading some medical literature—but no real explanation. The only thing I could tell her was that I was very hurt, and that I will not attend another psychiatrist, as all I learned about how to live and love was from you. This no one can take from me—not even a mother superior! . . . I feel so afraid and alone. . . . I'm sorry, Doctor, that you have to suffer the pain of this injustice. But know that there are many, many religious who would never question your competence despite what my superior has done.

Another religious flooded us with many, many desperate letters, including copies of her letters to the superior. Every one of the patients reacted in her own way; this one was the most outspoken. Fortunately, she was at that stage of therapy where she could turn the situation to her advantage by applying what she had learned about believing in herself, and asserting herself. In letters to her superior she wrote:

> Please tell me why you wish me to change to a new doctor now? You have me most bewildered after all the fine things you have always told me about my doctor. And I have personally concluded from my contacts with him that he is not only most competent, but also consistent and principled. He is the doctor I trust to leave—myself having grown to independent maturity, not with fear or "pining". . . It was through him and his influence alone that I am convinced I've begun to find God again, that I still want to be a religious woman as I've vowed and committed myself forever to be . . . Since I am the one with the emotional problem—and who wouldn't have emotional

problems after the training and treatment I've received and seen so many others receive in religious life—shouldn't I be the best qualified to judge as to whether or not I am receiving the competent guidance I need to achieve my goal—arrival at personal integrity? . . . You've taken the one kind, trustworthy, knowledgeable person I've been permitted to meet out of my life, and done it most brutally. Your action was not motherly, not professional, or sisterly! The trauma of all this is next to intolerable. You might as well have me shot by a firing squad . . . I fully realize what a debt I am to the congregation, and I was feeling guilty enough once to offer to repay my debts by temporarily leaving the order and finding gainful employment. I know my hospital stay was expensive, but it was also the turning point of my life. I was more relaxed after the insulin treatments, able to open up to the doctor, and I began sleeping so much better. The doctor warned me that the aftermath would not be easy as my tied-up feelings would slowly unwind more and more, and that there would be a seeming relapse. And he was right, the suffering has been acute, emotionally and physically, but before I went to the hospital, I was entirely sleepless, working around the clock in order to avoid having to face all my fears of everything and everyone.

All of these patients were affected for many months by anxiety and panic states, a return of many of their original complaints and symptoms, and a deep sense of loss toward their order which for some may well prove to be permanent.

### SPIRITUAL AFFIRMATION

In this chapter we have discussed the deprivation neurotic's response to and need for emotional and intellectual affirmation. It is only proper to briefly comment on the need for and effect

of spiritual affirmation if we may call so what is meant by the
"laying on of hands" or the "praying over a person" by others.
The reports of happenings in pentecostal prayer meetings and
charismatic communities which bring to mind the miraculous
cures reported in the Scriptures, are stimulating our scientific
curiosity to examine additional motives for considering the
significance of man's spiritual life on his whole being. Although
objective scientific studies of these reported charismatic heal-
ings—physical, emotional, mental and spiritual—are, as far as we
know, virtually non-existent, the writings of Agnes Sanford,
Kathryn Kuhlman, Rev. Francis MacNutt, O.P., and others, are
sufficiently persuasive to warrant in-depth investigation. In fact,
only by including such investigations in its approach to its
studies of man, can psychiatry be truly said to give due consideration to the whole man.

All we want to state on this subject, and that very briefly,
is that man's natural, undisturbed development from birth can
be described as a gradual growing on the three levels of his existence, the somatic, psychic (mental) and spiritual levels. With
the passage of time each "higher" level, provided it receives the
proper "nourishment," develops and becomes integrated with
the previous or "lower" level. The essential link between the
somatic and psychic levels consists of the sensory and emotional
life, that between the psychic and spiritual levels of the "super-
intellectual" infusion of faith and hope. To say it differently, on
the cognitive level the mature man functions by means of his
senses, intellect and faith, while he strives by means of his emotional love, will and hope.

No one disputes that soma and psyche influence each other
for better and for worse (psychosomatic illnesses). It is to be
expected that the same may well hold true for the psyche and
spirit of man. It is this aspect that we have touched upon earlier,
and will illustrate with some case histories, in discussing the
impact of both affirmation and denial on a person's religious
attitudes. There seems to be a growing body of evidence that

it is possible for a person's underdeveloped emotional life to grow and become integrated with his psyche (intellect and will), as well as for his disturbed thinking processes to return to normal, as the result of what might be called a proper stimulation of his spiritual life. Such spiritual affirmation, for instance, by the laying on of hands by persons whose faith and spiritual life are rich and overflowing, is reported to have resulted in improvement, if not cure, of neurotic and psychotic disorders. It is interesting to note that as the result of such "spiritual stimulation" many physical disorders—cancers, bone deformities, cardiovascular diseases, even congenital dental anomalies are commonly healed in a very short time, frequently overnight, while emotional and mental disorders seem to be resolved gradually and in stages, at intervals of days and weeks, if not longer, and only after repeated prayers and laying on of hands.

There is much that is still unclear and confused—in part undoubtedly as the result of semantics—in the realm of healing through prayer. However, there seems to be little that cannot be clarified, short of what always will remain a mystery defying all scientific investigation, by objective studies, free from emotional or philosophical prejudice, and guided by a sincere and fearless desire for greater knowledge of man even as this involves "suprahuman" powers.

Our greater ability to distinguish now more clearly between repressive neuroses, deprivation neuroses and schizophrenia may be considered a positive factor in any future scientific research of spiritual healing processes. Such research demands among other things that we can determine as clearly and scientifically as possible what kind of emotional or mental illness responds to prayer, under what circumstances on the part of the patient and the members of the praying community, by what psychological process, and what knowledge is required on the part of the "healer" about psychological and psychiatric matters in general, and about the individual patient's status in particular.

In our opinion it could well be, in fact it is something to be hoped for in our psychiatric specialty, "the chaotic, undisciplined discipline,"[3] that combined research by various members of the healing professions will make available a much more profound insight into the origin of man, his ultimate destination and the universal ingredients for his happiness.

1—The concept of affirmation is much more complex than it seems at first glance. It is *not* something a person *does* to another. Rather it is a state of *being*, of being aware and moved by the goodness of another being, which state is revealed without doing anything if the emotional life is fully developed and not repressed. For a more detailed discussion see *Born Only Once* by C. W. Baars, M.D.

2—Throughout this book, we have been careful to use the word "feel" solely in the literal sense of the word. That is to say, it cannot be equated with "think," as is done—unfortunately—more and more in present-day colloquial use. For instance, it is common to hear such expressions as, I *feel* that the law should be changed," or, "My broker *feels* that the stock market is too high," or, "Don't you *feel* that this war is immoral?", even though it must be clear to anyone that such statements, if they are to carry any weight in a discussion, must result from thinking and judging, not from feelings.

3—Enoch Callaway, M.D. in *Psychiatry Today*, April 1975.

# CHAPTER VII

# AFFIRMATION IN THERAPY AND DAILY LIFE

## LOVE AND TENDERNESS

The fact that the deprivation neurotic patient has to grow emotionally demands, in many severe cases, that he must experience the feelings of love and tenderness which were denied him in infancy. This is particularly true for female patients and, in most cases, an absolute requirement for their successful treatment. Male patients who were deprived of motherly tenderness also require maternal love and affection, but the tactile manifestations of this love—at least in our experience—play much less of a role. Young men often find such manifestations offensive to their feelings of manliness. On the other hand, they do desire expressions of affection in the form of cordiality, dedication, a warm interest in their welfare, and such exchanges of greetings and ways of relating as are customarily exhibited, for example, among men in Spain and Italy. We have seen several young men who were deprived of all motherly tenderness as children, but in therapy progressed well beyond these infantile needs without receiving any tactile expressions of tenderness. This difference between men and women is well demonstrated in the following case. We treated a young man with a typical deprivation neurosis. He had been living in a state of lasting depression, but we were able to help him a good deal, and we also placed him in a very friendly and cordial family where he could play with small children as much as he wanted. Recently he wrote that every

day in this home was a treat for him. Later, a younger sister of
his entered therapy. Brought up in the same psychically traumatic atmosphere, she had developed a severe deprivation neurosis. In her case all therapy proved vain until she received tactile
manifestations of motherly tenderness.

### NEED FOR TRUE LOVE IN FEMALE PATIENTS

The question of decisive importance in many cases, therefore,
is whether there is a person from whom the patient can receive
this feeling of love. There has to be someone who, first of all,
really possesses motherly affection for the patient, and, secondly,
is ready and willing to give expression to this feeling and to treat
the patient more or less as a child.

Such a person must have a genuine maternal feeling for the
patient. For it is not a matter of the patient merely receiving
tactile gratification. She desires and needs tactile expressions that
stem from *authentic love*. She needs these because, first of all,
she requires affirmation, the feeling that she is accepted and that
she is unique and worthwhile to another human being. But tactile sensations only convey this meaning when they proceed
from true feelings of love on the part of the person who provides them. One could say that these tactile stimulations, together
with the feelings of love, must constitute a *psychomotor whole*.
If a person caresses a girl solely for the purpose of helping her,
as a therapeutic gesture without a feeling of real love, the intended effect will definitely not occur. A sensitive patient will
immediately feel that the caress is not prompted by true love,
and consequently it is deprived of any curative action. Besides,
there is something dishonest about giving someone certain expressions of tenderness when they are not the result of love for
her. It means that one wants her to feel a love which actually
does not exist! Of course, if this loves does exist, it should be
expressed to help the other. What does matter is that such expressions should truly correspond with the feelings of the persons who show them.

In recent years much has been written about man's need for love. Weekend courses show people how to free their emotions through *sensitivity training;* even religious gatherings are held with this goal in mind; in some places psychotherapeutic sessions are conducted in the nude to free the participants from emotional inhibitions. We do not intend to discuss here the pros and cons of such gatherings, which are not always professionally conducted or motivated. We only want to illustrate the dangers which are incurred by going through the motions of loving a patient without having any real feeling for him, even when such a pretense is motivated by the most sincere desire to help. The following case is even more noteworthy in this connection because the *techniques* were applied to a male patient, and the needs of men, as we shall discuss later on in this chapter, differ from those of women. We quote excerpts from a letter written by the patient, a middle-aged, unmarried, professional man who had been unable to perform his duties for some time, due to a most disabling deprivation neurosis and to an equally severe superimposed fear neurosis.

> Dear Doctor: What a terrible week this has been; I feel awful, worse than usual. I can't cope with life, and it is worse since this incident. The social worker I've told you about came to see me. He had been to some kind of a seminar on sensitivity, and he began to try on me some of the things he had learned. He started out by saying, "I love you," and things like that. Also "You are a great guy." I told him I did not believe that. He replied that I needed to love and be loved, and the only way I could do this was by going out and meet people and be with people. I told him that he knew how scared I was of everybody. He said I could stop going to the doctor if I followed his advice, as I would be cured. He kept repeating how he loved me until I started to cry because his insistence scared me to death. While I was crying he embraced me and ran his hand through my hair. I did not

like this at all, but I was too scared to tell him so. After all he meant so well, and I did not want to hurt his feelings. But I felt like he was trying to make me do something I was not ready for. I also felt he was experimenting on me. The effects of this session were most disturbing to me. The next day he returned for more of the same. I got up to leave the room, but he started to chase me. I finally escaped and locked myself in the bathroom. For a while he kept it up through the closed door, but finally left. I was all upset about his attack on me, and I still tremble at the memory. I used to trust him, and intellectually I know he means well and has no ulterior motives. But now I cannot trust him anymore, or feel secure with him as I did before. Now you are the only one left I can trust. Please do not give up on me.

It is necessary, therefore, that there be somebody who really loves the patient. This person, of course, must be someone who is older than the patient, and preferably a woman, so that her love for the patient can have something maternal in it.

Furthermore, the person who really loves the patient must be willing to give expression to her feelings for the patient and to treat the patient more or less as a child. To do so has definite consequences, for once this relationship has been entered into, the manifestations of love result in an even stronger union. To do otherwise, to loosen this bond after some time, hurts the patient in the deepest and most vulnerable aspects of her life. By such an action the patient feels abandoned and, indeed, is pushed deeper into her neurosis. For until then the patient has come to believe that she is worth loving, and now suddenly she experiences, at least in her feelings, that this is not so. And since she experiences this from the person to whom she has surrendered herself and who knows her innermost thoughts and feelings, she cannot but arrive at the conclusion that she is not worth loving. The affirmation which the patient had received from the other person's maternal tenderness and affection becomes the opposite—rejection, denial.

Possession of this maternal love also requires that one care for the patient in a motherly fashion. Emotionally, the patient experiences her relationship with the other person as a mother-child relationship, and accordingly expects from it everything which such a relationship entails. In reality her expectations in this regard cannot be fully materialized, for the simple reason that the other person is not actually her mother and can never completely satisfy her desires. The patient will not be hurt as long as she is denied this satisfaction for an adequate reason, for she can understand why this has to be so and will accept it. But the patient should be given whatever is reasonable. The foster mother will have to help her and take care of her, and tolerate her peculiarities, just as a real mother does with her own child. If the foster mother really loves the girl, she will be pleased to do these things with real dedication; nor will it be a heavy burden because her love will lighten the task.

As a consequence of the fact that the person who shows this motherly affection to the patient is not really her mother, *manifestations of tender affection must remain within proper bounds.* Otherwise, there will be danger that the patient, whose reason cannot provide the necessary inhibitions, will demand too much, for the unrestrained gratification of her desires might jeopardize the proper relationship.

It is not uncommon for deprivation neurotic girls to long for the mother's breast and want to drink from it like a baby. One day a woman, approximately forty-five years of age and a resident of another country, came to us for advice. She was not married, but had assumed the care of a young girl who had been abandoned by her own mother and never received motherly love and affection. Over the years the girl had become very attached to this woman and felt toward her like a real daughter. When the younger woman developed a desire to drink from her breast, the woman had consented but became doubtful whether she had done the right thing, both morally and mentally. We were able to put her mind at ease about the moral aspect, as it was evident that she had acted with the purest intentions. In regard to the mental aspect, we pointed out that giving the breast means feeding in both an essential and a biological sense. Since in this case there was no question of feeding, the act represented something untrue and for this reason we could not consider it right. However, as long as she had started, it would not be right to discontinue the practice abruptly. Sometime later the woman wrote to inform us that the girl had outgrown the practice spontaneously. In all cases of deprivation neurotic patients who tell of experiencing a desire to drink from the breasts of their foster mothers, we have always presented this same explanation to show why the foster mother cannot satisfy their desire. All these patients have been able to accept this reason without it being an obstacle to their emotional growth in therapy.[1]

Sometimes patients desire even more than this. They wish to be reborn physically from their foster mother. Since this is obviously impossible, the foster mother can explain to the girl that such an act is not necessary and that through her love she gives new life, causing the patient to experience something even more important, namely, her *second birth* or *psychic incarnation.*

### NEED FOR TRUE LOVE IN MALE PATIENTS

If young men with a deprivation neurosis are in need of motherly tenderness, it is sometimes possible that an older woman with maternal feelings toward them can help. Such a woman has to be older and must be absolutely emotionally mature. These two requirements are even more necessary here than in the case of girl patients, for although these young men may be psychologically retarded, they are physically adult and therefore exposed to the danger that tactile manifestations of affection may arouse other feelings which are incompatible with the actual relationship.

Later in therapy the need for motherly affection is often

supplemented by the need for fatherly concern and help. Affirmation by a father figure is of particular importance in the case of male patients, for, as we have said before, they often need this kind of affirmation more than motherly tenderness. They need to experience the firm support and steadfastness of the father through his words, understanding, and manly cordiality.

Still, female patients too may feel a need for fatherly care and concern. It hardly needs repeating that in these cases also the proper relationship must be preserved carefully, and the father figure, as far as his feelings and conduct are concerned, must remain a father at all times. If he were to lose sight of the need to preserve this relationship, the consequences would be disastrous for the girl involved. Although the female deprivation neurotic may feel like a child, she is physically full-grown and capable of developing the feelings of an adult woman. Our warning about manifestations of tactile tenderness for a male patient by an older and more mature woman applies in these cases *a fortiori*.

### PLAY

Important as sensitive love and affection are for the total development of every human being, still other factors contribute to the development of man's emotional life. A child likes and needs to play, and the various forms of play help him to grow emotionally. The same process of emotional growth through play is often observed in the therapy of deprivation neurotic individuals.

Female patients, for example, may get the desire to play with a *teddy bear and dolls*. Interestingly enough, the desire for the teddy bear or some other toy animal comes first. The desire for a doll comes later and is a step forward in the growing process. This sequence is natural. Following a period of playing in the sandbox, during which the child familiarizes himself with a non-living, physical substance and makes it submit to his will, the animal, which nature has ordained to be subordinate to man, presents itself to the child. The human being is next, but first under the image of the doll which, being completely docile, permits the child a sense of being superior. This play prepares the way to the child's contact with his peers and after this with grown-ups.

In the first five years of our psychiatric practice we never observed a male patient develop this desire to play with a teddy bear. This inclined us to think that playing with teddy bears presented a typical feminine characteristic. But then teddy bears suddenly played an important role in the development of the emotional life of two male patients.

The first case was that of a young man who told us one day: "If you ever want me for something, Doctor, go downtown to any of the stores where they sell teddy bears. I simply can't tear myself away from those places." When we asked him why he didn't buy himself a teddy bear, he replied, "But isn't that silly?" Months later he finally dared to buy one and told us how much happiness he derived from looking at the bear when studying at his desk in the evening; it was better than listening to the radio. The teddy bear dispelled the feeling of loneliness that was always with him in his bachelor living quarters. But later, when, with difficulty and reluctance, he told his fiancée about the teddy bear, she laughed at him, and called him a childish fellow. He was hurt so deeply by this reply, which indicated that she had failed to understand the meaning of his delicate feeling toward the teddy bear, that it affected his love for her. This incident led to the breaking of the engagement—which, incidentally, was a good thing, for they were not at all suited to each other.

The other case was that of a medical student who, in a sudden need to pour out his heart, disclosed: "Doctor, I have committed the worst deed of my life. I have burned the teddy bear of my childhood. I have hurt myself deeply by doing this, I'm afraid." It appeared that he had saved the teddy bear through the years until one day he said to himself, "Be a man and throw that thing away." Without further thought he had pulled off the legs and burned the whole thing. It was suggested that he buy another bear, but he felt that it would be of no use since a new teddy bear could never be the one of his childhood.[2]

The majority of young men and boys, however, develop a desire for *physical achievements,* participation in various sports, technical hobbies, handicrafts, electric trains, photography, and other pastimes. We remember seeing a cartoon of a heavy-set man sitting on the floor of his living room playing with his son's electric train. The boy is standing nearby watching his father and asks: "Dad, are you playing in earnest, or is this merely a repressed complex?" If the cartoonist had been familiar with the syndrome of deprivation neurosis, the caption might well have read: "Dad, are you playing in earnest, or do you have a deprivation neurosis?"

Frequently it is quite important for male patients to have the opportunity to play and romp with boys in such a way that they can forget themselves and behave as befits their mental age, unencumbered by the fact that their chronological age far exceeds their psychological stage of development. Earlier we mentioned the case of an adult male patient whose emotional life unfolded and matured only after he had made his home with a warm and friendly family and could take part in games with the children. Another patient, a psychology major at a university, once asked for permission to be admitted to an institution for the psychotherapy of children. In that way, he thought, he would be able to play as a boy with the other boys and thus would progress considerably in his emotional growth. Another patient, a professional man, was absolutely incapable of performing the duties of his state. When we succeeded in getting him the position of supervisor in an orphanage for boys, he had the opportunity to participate in all their activities. This did him a lot of good and enhanced his progress considerably. The only thing he had to watch out for, he told us, was that he could not permit himself to quarrel with the boys, although he was often greatly tempted to do so. Occasionally, the tendency to want to romp with boys is suspected of having a sexual element. This, it must be stated emphatically, is not true for patients who suffer solely from a deprivation neurosis. What matters in their case is that they have an opportunity to express themselves spontaneously, precisely as they feel, that is, as a child.

A remarkable example of this childish mentality was the case of a medical specialist whose wife came to us for advice because she had been worried about him for a long time. She began by saying that he was a good man, but that at times he acted strangely, almost like a child. For instance, when walking in the yard not long before, she had suddenly seen her husband on the roof of their house. Later, when she had asked him what kind of trouble had made him climb onto the roof, he laughingly replied that there was no trouble, but he had thought it would be fun to climb onto the roof. On his birthday he had put the presents which he had received on a bench in front of the fireplace. These were a tube of toothpaste, a saucer with oranges from the grocer, and, on another plate, some money allegedly from his father. At some other time in the past, when their six-year-old son had received a toy train for a present, she had found her husband absorbed in playing with it one evening after the boy had gone to bed. His wife also told us that each time he visited with one of the neighbors, the latter's eight-year-old son took off in tears because her husband always picked a fight with him. There were still other observations which made it not at all difficult to make a diagnosis of deprivation neurosis. The accounts due him for professional services amounted to thousands of dollars simply because he did not dare to send out statements to his patients. His wife tried to do this herself even though this often led to arguments between them. And as soon as anybody made the slightest objection to the amount of his bill, the physician tore it up at once and dropped the whole matter. The explanation of this kind of behavior is both simple and typical of deprivation neurotics: fear of displeasing others. Furthermore, this man blamed himself for everything that went wrong. If one of his patients got worse instead of better, he would break and destroy something because he reproached himself for the patient's condition and was afraid that the relatives of the patient would blame him. And if one of his patients died, he would send flowers in order to make up for his guilt. Again, these are the frustration neurotic's typical feelings of inadequacy and guilt.

### CHILDISH DESIRES

It is the task of the therapist to guide the developing childish desires of patients. The therapist must encourage patients as much as possible without showing any sign of disapproval or surprise. Naturally, what these patients desire cannot compare with the desires of a mature adult, but this the therapist understands. He knows that his patients are not that far as yet in their development, and that these *childish gratifications are necessary* for the growth of their emotional lives. The fact that he completely agrees with and shows a sincere interest in these childish joys is an important source of affirmation for the patients. They need this affirmation, for they usually realize full well that their desires are childish and immature. The affirmation of the therapist makes it possible for them to give in freely to their desires. This attitude on the part of the therapist is different from that he must show toward patients suffering from a repressive neurosis. In those patients, he let the repressed material be discharged without encouragement on his part. In deprivation neurotic patients, however, whenever possible, he promotes the growth of the emotions in a positive manner.

Whether it is possible to gratify these childish desires depends, as we mentioned earlier, largely on the circumstances of each case. For instance, many healthy desires cannot be gratified when the necessary financial means are lacking. In such cases one can only try to do what is possible, and for the rest must wait and see what will come of it. Normally, human nature helps us to overcome the various less favorable factors in our environment. This also happens in the therapeutic situation, provided that there exists a sound natural drive toward healthy development. The situation is analogous to physical illness, in which a cure often depends on the person's *driving force toward health.*

If this force is absent, as occurs in an asthenic personality, who by himself possesses little or no stimulus to forge ahead, then the reaction to disappointments is often a severe depression.

The therapist, therefore, as much as is in his power, must first promote the psychic development of his patient by trying to help him gratify those desires which are proper to his childish level of development. Also, he must keep this development within reasonable limits by trying to prevent everything that would be unreasonable and, thus, harmful to his patient's emotional development. For instance, it may happen that certain desires could cause a conflict between the patient and his environment. To give but one example, if a patient with a deprivation neurosis is entirely dependent on his job for his existence and develops infantile desires which if expressed would jeopardize his job, he should be advised to desist from these desires for his own sake. Or when parents or relatives disapprove of certain things and the patient is financially dependent on them, he would be wise to give up those things, for otherwise his situation will get worse.

### INTEGRATION OF EMOTIONS AND REASON

Although we have stressed the need for the patient to grow emotionally, we must not forget that there must also be an accompanying infiltration of reason into his emotional life such as occurs in every normal human being. Obviously a deprivation neurotic patient cannot bring this about immediately; in this way, too, he is like a pre-adolescent whose parents have to provide him with the norms for his actions as long as reason and emotion do not operate together harmoniously. If the therapist fails in his duty to do the same for his patient and gives him license to do as he pleases, the patient is in danger of becoming fixed in a state of emotional semi-maturity, of being like a spoiled child. Such tragic development, or rather lack of development, shows itself in the fact that such patients do not learn to respect other people or to take their feelings into consideration in a mature, non-fearful fashion. Like the pre-adolescent, their interest remains centered on themselves. The *therapist must provide intelligent guidance* in this stage of growth and help patients to *form sound judgments without distortion of their feelings.* If for the moment his efforts would be in vain, the therapist has no choice but to tolerate the consequences. He can only hope that at some future time he will be able to give his patient a proper insight into the nature of his feelings.

### PSYCHOSEXUAL DEVELOPMENT

Sexuality is an aspect of the therapeutic guidance of these patients which often presents special difficulties. Their condition in this regard is most peculiar. Physically and sexually they are fully grown in every respect, which means that they are subject to the influence of the sex hormones. The psychic aspect of their sexuality, however, is far from fully grown and this is especially true for the integration of their sexuality into their love for another person. One might well say that the sexual act, if it is part of their life, has an exclusively organic, non-psychic character. Such patients perform or endure the sexual act without experiencing a meaningful psychic relation with the partner, without giving themselves to the other. One of our patients had lived with a young man before she entered therapy. Circumstances had led to this intimate relationship between them, but she herself had never been emotionally involved to any extent, nor had she developed any special attachment for the young man. In spite of their close physical relationship, she was not emotionally involved at all.

The incidence of *masturbation* in young men with this type of neurosis is, as far as we can determine, neither more nor less than in individuals who are not deprivation neurotics. The influence of continuing growth toward physical maturity, which in puberty gives rise to masturbation, makes itself felt equally in persons with or without this neurosis. The only difference is that the imagination, which under normal circumstances becomes spontaneously directed at another person, does not do so in these patients. In some of our patients, masturbation did not develop until their late twenties or middle thirties.

When young men with a deprivation neurosis come in contact with girls, they often look only for tenderness. This becomes a source of bitter disappointment for the girl since she is not aware that the young man merely desires motherly tenderness and she experiences her relation as a normally erotic one. In the meantime, her emotions develop into feelings of love which, she suddenly discovers, the other does not reciprocate.[3]

Men with a deprivation neurosis not infrequently seek contact with *prostitutes*, albeit in a peculiar fashion insofar as these contacts seldom reach the point of intercourse. It is our impression that curiosity motivates many of these men. Also, they have the desire to be accepted by another person in everything, no matter what their inner feelings and disposition.

In a few cases, deprivation neurotic patients have told us of having *exhibitionistic* tendencies or having engaged in exhibitionist acts. But instead of being driven by sexual desires, these patients were merely moved by the wish to draw attention to themselves and to be fully accepted by others.

*Homosexual* acts, too, may occur. In the cases of the deprivation neurotics which we have studied personally, the basic motive always appeared to be the fact that the missing motherly tendencies in childhood had made it impossible for them to feel that a woman was something good, an object toward which their feelings could be directed. Consequently, their feelings, including the sexual ones, had been directed at an object of the same sex. In several of our cases the homosexual orientation disappeared when the neurosis was cured, making room for a normal heterosexual orientation which enabled the patient to enter into a sound and happy marriage relationship.

In girls the sexual development is often insignificant. Masturbation frequently does not occur at all. But since girls do have an intense need for love and tenderness, it sometimes happens that they too are accused of being homosexual. This is not so strange, for it is to be expected that only a woman can give them the tenderness they desire so much. And if they do establish a close tie with another girl or woman, this relationship is often interpreted as being homosexual. These patients come to us repeatedly because they are afraid that they might be homosexuals or because others have said this of them, even though there has never been any sexual contact, but only a strong mutual love. This, of course, has nothing to do with homosexuality. All they want is tenderness.

One of our patients was a married woman and the mother of several children. Her married life gave her little satisfaction; she experienced sexual relations with her husband in a dutiful manner but without any participation of her feelings. Because she had a great need for friendship with girls, her husband had begun to suspect her of homosexuality and was contemplating divorce. It soon became clear that this woman was not at all a homosexual but did suffer from a deprivation neurosis. Having been deprived of tender love in childhood, she had come to seek this from girls with whom there had never been any sexual contact. We explained her condition to her and showed how this need had grown. We made it clear that no homosexuality was involved, and that she should not consider her feelings wrong but rather should experience them quietly. A great calm came over her when she understood the nature of her feelings and allowed herself to live accordingly. Eventually her feelings unfolded in their strength, including those toward her husband, and thus divorce was averted.

Another example is a girl who was referred to us by a priest because she had developed a friendly relationship with one of his female penitents and wanted much tenderness from her. The priest, thinking that she was a homosexual, wanted to protect his penitent from difficulties and with her permission suggested to the girl that she seek our advice. She appeared to be a fine, sensitive girl with normal muscle stretch reflexes but with an uncomplicated and not too severe deprivation neurosis. She had no need for sexual gratification but had become confused when the priest had begun to suspect her of being homosexual. Fortunately, both the priest and his penitent accepted my explanation of the situation and agreed to continue the relationship. At the time of writing this book, five years after this incident, it can be reported that no sexual relations of any kind ever occurred between these two women. The girl we saw in consultation has matured to a normal loving woman; she is happily married to a widower with five young children.

When the emotional life of such patients develops properly, their egocentricity recedes gradually, and as feelings for other people develop, they often begin, as is to be expected, to feel love for a person of the opposite sex. This is, of course, an ordinary symptom which sooner or later will manifest itself. Sometimes this occurs without any special difficulties, whether the patient is still single and entirely free, or when he is married or living under solemn vows. If the patients are single, they have the prospect of a good engagement period followed by a happy marriage, provided they await the proper moment to take this step. How important this is we were able to observe in the case of a young man and a girl who both had a deprivation neurosis. Twice they became engaged and twice they broke it off. The third time, five years later, they were able to really love each other, and everything went smoothly from there on. If the patients are already married and have had the opportunity to make up for the insufficient development which existed at the time the marriage took place, the marriage has an excellent chance to become a happy one. This happened in the previously discussed case of the woman who did not want a child during the first five years of her marriage, but preferred to play with a doll. Her understanding husband respected her condition patiently. Eventually she matured so much in therapy that she wanted a child. On the arrival of the baby their family life became entirely normal.

If patients live under vows, a thorough therapy will enable them to accept their state of life with firm conviction and wholehearted dedication and to live happily as priest, monk, brother, or nun. Some of them then experience a need to take their vows anew, because the first ones, taken under different emotional conditions, no longer possess value in their eyes.

These are the fortunate cases. But things can be quite different. To reach the stage of being able to experience love for another may be a source of considerable difficulties. For instance, a patient may fall in love with someone who does not reciprocate this love. If this is a most painful experience for normal young people, the consequences are much more serious for persons with a deprivation neurosis. At such a time they are suddenly affirmed again in their feelings of inferiority and in their opinion that they are unworthy of being loved. This can impede the recovery process considerably.

If the patients are married, it may become evident that at the time of marriage there existed no real love for the partner, only a childish affection. Under such circumstances there often exists no other choice, especially if there are children to be considered, than to accept the marriage as it is, with all the difficulties a loveless union entails.

If the patients are bound by vows and their development in therapy does not lead to a mature acceptance of what they had chosen when still immature, different courses of action may be followed. In the case of a religious nun or a lay brother, there would be ample reason to dispense them of their vows. It is only reasonable not to want to hold a person for life to a state which he chose without sufficient emotional integrity. In the case of a priest, it would seem, at least from a psychiatric viewpoint, that dispensation from the vow of celibacy would also be the proper solution. Be that as it may, it does not belong to our field of competency to judge the correctness of such a step. At any rate, in all such cases the psychotherapist will have to be a source of lasting support to his patients. He must show them the correct way and make it possible for them, through his moral support and cordial interest, to go forward on their journey through life.

One more point remains to be discussed about the development of the deprivation neurotic patient, namely, his attitude toward religion. Generally speaking, religion means nothing to him. This is not difficult to understand. The exercise of true religion is, in essence, the act of a mature, adult individual. It is an attitude toward the ultimate goal of existence, and presumes a psychic being in which the spiritual dominates and the sensitive is subject to the spiritual, always a hallmark of real maturity. The religion of children is a spontaneous expression of their feelings, just as everything in nature is directed to its ultimate goal. In the normal development of a person, this childish expression, which is predominantly sensitive, grows along with the emotional life and becomes integrated harmoniously with the intellect.

This harmonious development does not take place in deprivation neurotics, however, because the growth of the emotional life is arrested early while the intellect continues to grow and leaves the feelings far behind. Consequently, the childish religious feelings in these patients disappear because they are proportionate to a child's knowledge, while mature religious feeling, which corresponds to an increased knowledge of spiritual matters, cannot develop. It is not surprising then that religious spiritual values and, indeed, corresponding religious practices have little or no meaning for deprivation neurotics and do not appeal to their feelings. Such individuals simply have not reached a stage at which religious values can attract them. As a result, the practices that these values entail are easily neglected, and if they are kept up through the years, it is because the individual feels more or less coerced to maintain the practices, often experiencing a great sense of relief when such customs are finally abandoned. However, it should not be concluded that these persons have no faith left and are no longer religious. Their fundamental orientation toward God remains unchanged, but the external acknowledgement of this belief has become an impossibility for them.

One need not worry in the least about the temporary abandonment of religious practices among these neurotics when in therapy. At the proper time their orientation toward God will come spontaneously to the surface, and they will begin to acknowledge externally what has been present interiorly all along. Especially as they experience the love which they need so very much for the growth of their emotional life, their religious life opens up again. We are acquainted with numerous individuals who had neglected their religion completely for many years, but during therapy for their deprivation neurosis spontaneously resumed the practice of religious duties, and, in the case of Catholics, even became daily communicants. But this happens only when they can see their religion for what it really is, or at least what it should be: namely, the experiencing of the love of God and of love for God. Like all human beings, these individuals want love not only in their natural lives, but also in their supernatural life with God.

For this reason it is a most regrettable thing that the Catholic Church, at least as she often appears to the outside world, seems incapable of attracting these patients, but rather repels them by not offering them an affirmation of their whole being. They are frightened by the complex of legal commandments, threats, and punishments by which the Church is often, in their eyes, characterized, while God is felt as a threatening, powerful force. From all sides, they feel overwhelmed by demands and isolated in their weakness, uncertainty, and feelings of guilt.

A paragraph from a patient's letter may serve as an example of this; it was written by a woman with a severe deprivation neurosis who even as a child was overcome by fear of God. "My inner fear has taken on form from what I heard about God. It was always God who made things wrong, who made it possible to do things wrong. More and more, things were turned into threats by God. My only purpose in life was to keep things

right in the eyes of God." This woman was known to us as a
deeply religious person, but the thought of God always aroused
her fears; she simply could not bear to think of Him or to hear
about Him. A case like this shows how the Church and religion
may become a source of intense fear if the real truths about the
Church and religion are not made known in the proper manner
or at the proper time. But the real Church, the Church of Love,
the Church of Christ, always attracts. One never has to be afraid
to tell patients of the truths which proclaim this love and reveal
Christ's goodness and tenderness, for these truths open their
souls and enable them to live in confidence and joy.[4]

## EMOTIONAL GROWTH IN THERAPY

The patient has to overcome all these various difficulties if
he is to grow and develop gradually through the various phases
of psychic life, thus compensating for his retarded development.
The more he grows, the more the symptoms of his illness—the
uncertainties, fears, and feelings of inferiority—disappear. One
must not forget, however, that these feelings and fears have had
ample opportunity to anchor themselves in the patient's emotional life during the many years that he had to live with his
neurosis. Consequently, it will always take considerable time
before they can be mobilized and lose the firm hold they have
obtained over the years, in order to make room for normal
emotional reactions. In these difficult years, the therapist has the
none-too-easy task of accompanying the patient on the long
road to recovery; listening to him again and again, reassuring
and affirming him repeatedly. For the most part, therapy consists of creating an atmosphere in which the patient feels calm
and safe, and which serves as a never ending source of the courage and strength he needs to continue on the difficult path
toward recovery.

It cannot be denied that this path is difficult for deprivation
neurotics. They become increasingly aware of how little they
are suited for the life they have to lead and how much patience

and faith they need in order to persevere. Much *patience* is necessary to withstand the repeated disappointments, the unavoidable setbacks, the mistaken judgments of their condition and the criticism to which they are frequently exposed. They must learn to see these painful experiences as relative and transient in character and thus unable to prevent their cure and growth to maturity. It takes much confidence to be optimistic about the future and recovery, yet without this confidence patients could not keep going. As long as there is hope that they can outgrow their unhappy state, however, they can endure many things. For this reason the therapist must resolve all their doubts and despairs about their future, and show them repeatedly that it is possible to compensate for retarded growth. Whenever possible, he must show them in what way they have already made progress. The importance of this is seen when, as a result of unfortunate circumstances, progress does not take place, and the patient then experiences the greatest difficulty in trying to keep going.

This all becomes more clear as one reads the following letter. It was written by a man who gave up his medical studies because of a severe deprivation neurosis and then tried to support himself in a job for which he was ill-equipped emotionally. These and many other disappointments finally culminated in the rejection he experienced when the girl he loved did not return his affection.

> Dear Doctor: What infinite patience is required in order to accept all these things! One has to overlook so many things that hurt. There are so many wishes that never come true. Sometimes the disappointments are so painful.
>
> It is impossible for me to be outgoing; I cannot be interested in others. I feel so ill at ease and inadequate in the many and varied relationships which exist among people. Should there not be some friendship, some emotional ties with a few persons? As a rule, I find myself outside of the group to which I belong. My remarks are ignored

and stir no response. When I speak to another, the conversation soon dies. It is only by means of generalities and platitudes that I can keep it going for a while. There seems to be no answer to all these things, at least not to me. Although I have not got to the point where I can accept this condition, at least I still have strength to bear it and to hold up under it. But a feeling of rebellion and bitterness creeps up in me because this condition has lasted so long and is so confusing. What is the sense and the ultimate meaning of it? I cannot help despairing for I see no way out.

This man, it must be added, was deeply religious. His surrender to God's providence finally gave him the courage to carry on.

It is a different matter for those who lack this strong supernatural faith; usually they develop the most serious depressions. If at all possible, the therapist must try to prevent such depressions. He must help his patients to take the proper attitude in regard to the recurring symptoms of their illnesses. For instance, he will help them to reduce their excessive eagerness to please others by making it clear that they are not selfish if they go their own way. He will help them to understand that it is not a sign of disordered love of self when they do not try to please others, and that they must learn not to submit to unreasonable fears of displeasing people. He will explain that they are going to feel uncomfortable no matter what they do. If patients are overly concerned about others, the fear of causing displeasure makes them act irrationally and feel ill at ease. If patients do what they know is right, they worry that the feelings of others will be hurt. The therapist must help his patients to *do what is right rather than try to please others*. He must approve their actions and help them to bear any unpleasant or disturbing feelings that result. He must absorb fears and make them bearable; he must offer courage when the patient has none and must allow angry outbursts to pass with sympathetic understanding. The therapist must take into account the capacities of each individual patient, and must never demand more than the patient can be expected to do. The patient must always feel safe with the therapist and know that the therapist will provide him with the necessary understanding and sympathy. Should it happen that the therapist has to refuse something, the patient will feel that this was only because the therapist loves him, is concerned for his welfare, and wants to protect him from possible harm.

Generally speaking, it is best for patients to have an attitude of *tolerance* toward their own shortcomings and defects, to endure them until they are outgrown. Patients must try to go against their inclination to hold themselves morally responsible for these shortcomings as best they can, and dare to believe that the disappearance of shortcomings is something which happens by itself during the period of psychic growth. To try to bring this about directly on his own is impossible and beyond the patient's power. Every attempt in this direction becomes a bitter disappointment, never failing to be a setback on the patient's path to recovery.

Such *setbacks*, by the way, whatever their cause, should never be a source of surprise to patients. Feelings of inadequacy and inferiority, morbid fear reactions, and all the other symptoms are rooted so deeply that it takes little in the way of unfavorable and emotionally traumatic circumstances to arouse them anew, even when the patients feel they are making excellent progress. As a matter of fact it is precisely during periods of actual emotional growth that setbacks are likely to occur. The reason for this is that the patients' subjective sense of well-being and greater emotional energy tempts them to again bend over backward to please others. The subsequent return of depression and other symptoms are good learning experiences and stimuli to resume their newly learned assertive behavior. But whatever the reasons for relapses the patients should be assured that they are no reason for concern and that the symptoms will eventually disappear by themselves. Symptoms, it should be explained, like so many tender spots remaining after a physical illness or an operation, may be aggravated occasionally before they disappear ultimately.[5]

### CHANGES IN COGNITION AND BEHAVIOR

Earlier, in the discussion of the symptomatology of the deprivation neurosis, we mentioned the abnormalities which may occur in the area of cognition and behavior. Nothing can be done to improve these defects, not even symptomatically. And if too much attention is paid to them, they only become worse. The thing to remember in this respect is that the cognitive life grows along with the emotional life, and as a result defects disappear spontaneously when patients grow emotionally.

Earlier, we pointed out the infantile aspect of the sensory perceptions of many deprivation neurotics. In this connection it is important to report what one of our patients wrote us about the evolution of her sense impressions:

> First of all, I want to tell you that my sense of taste has developed more. In the beginning I had an almost insatiable hunger for candy, especially candy that children prefer and not just for a few pieces but for a mouthful at a time. It was only very gradually that I began to long for something better, something more refined. At first I liked everything sweet, the sweeter the better; it did not matter what form it had, provided it was abundant. Things that tasted bitter I thought were horrible, while sour and salty things had little appeal for me.
>
> My indiscriminate craving for sweetness was followed by a preference for milk chocolate. Here again, the more the better, so that I could taste and feel it at the same time, so to speak; big pieces of milk chocolate I experienced as something good. After this, or rather in the meantime, I also began to appreciate something finer occasionally. My taste was not yet for more expensive bonbons or finest quality chocolate; in fact, I did not even

like those things and preferred a large piece or quantity of some ordinary candy.

Then suddenly I began to notice that my taste became more expensive; I began to prefer the better quality chocolate. And instead of quantity, I now began to put emphasis on quality. At present my taste appreciates most the finer delicacies so much so that it puts me in a happy mood. I find much pleasure in a fine bonbon and pastry, as well as in all kinds of dishes which my childish taste had led me to abhor. A glass of red wine is now a treat rather than a sour medicinal drink.

Until a relatively short time ago, I only liked the so-called sweet dishes such as applesauce and carrots, creamy and bland desserts, and the non-spiced soups. All this has changed. Asparagus, mushrooms, a spicy soup, tomatoes, an aged cheese, these and many other "adult" foods have my fullest attention and appreciation.

In retrospect, I realize that my sense of smell developed at the same time as my sense of taste. I never used eau de cologne, but now I have a real desire for it. The same is true for a good perfume; it can make me really happy. It seems to me that this sense is still in the process of further growth.

My sight and hearing are developing, too. I distinguish finer nuances in a voice. It is love that makes everything look and sound differently. A change of voice or facial expression is noticed immediately and tells me whether the other is happy or sad.

This interesting letter makes it clear that one has to wait patiently until the external and internal senses spontaneously grow and improve in their functioning. Nothing can be done to force this artificially. This is also true in the case of students who often have great difficulties with their *studies*. To force them to apply themselves in their studies at all costs makes no sense and will not improve their marks. The only thing which often helps is our aforementioned advice, to act as if the studies of these patients are play activities. In other words, they study without feeling that they have to, but because and to the extent that it interests them and gives them pleasure. By doing this, they are led by their feelings—precisely as children follow their feelings—and do not have to act like adults who do things in order to reach a goal. For the rest, one can only hope that an inner urge to study will become strong enough to enable them to persevere even when it is unpleasant to do so.

In general, it is wise not to be hasty in advising neurotic boys and girls with good innate intellects to change schools. It is usually better for them to continue in the school, college, or subject they have chosen, even though it may be necessary to repeat a grade or to get additional help with their studies. If they transfer to another school, the same difficulties will soon become manifest again, and it will then be even more difficult to adjust to a new environment than it would have been to remain in an old and familiar one.

### INSIGHT

One final remark remains to be made, a remark which perhaps would have been more suitable at the beginning. In order to make therapy at all possible, it will always be necessary to prepare the way by providing the patient with insight into his psychic condition. In practically all cases of deprivation neurosis, one is dealing with an intellectually adult individual who will never permit his emotional life to evolve unless he first understands the nature of his illness and realizes the necessity and reasonableness of accepting such evolution. In our experience, if the diagnosis is correct, the patient will have no difficulty in comprehending the therapist's explanation. In fact, after all the misery he usually has experienced, the patient will feel as though a heavy load is being lifted from his shoulders. It will be easier for him to judge and evaluate his inner life correctly and to see

it in the proper perspective. This by itself will do much to alleviate or at least diminish the burden under which he lives. And
what is most important of all, he will at last feel himself to be
understood by another person and, therefore, no longer alone.
This is truly an important factor in the affirmation of a person
with a deprivation neurosis.

"REVERSE FAMILY THERAPY"

We want to conclude these two chapters on therapy by
commenting briefly on a perhaps novel and different aspect of
therapy which may prove to be of some practical value even
though it is unlikely to find widespread application. Family
therapy, that is, the involvement of all members of a family in
the treatment of one of its sick members by one or more therapists or counselors is a well known treatment model. But the
reverse, so to speak, the treatment of one or more patients by a
therapist and his family is not. This novel "experiment" was
thrusted upon one of the authors when four of his patients in
an institute objected to the ways of its management and decided
to leave. This they did in spite of the fact that it would entail
separation from their therapist and their return home where no
other psychiatric therapy would be available than that which
had proved futile in the past.

Since they had been receiving affirmation therapy for several
months with noticeable improvement and a good prognosis
seemed likely if this therapy could be continued, their therapist,
after consulting with his wife and children, invited them to their
home for whatever length of time it would be necessary to
recover. Thus began an experiment in living and relating which
differed from the well known live-in arrangements for a mentally ill person in Gheel, Belgium, in that four patients received
almost daily therapy while living with their therapist and his
family, none of whom had ever been involved professionally with
emotionally ill persons. As the exposure to a normal, natural
family life was a totally new experience for all of them it seems

certain that it constituted a significant contribution to their
eventual recovery.

All four, two priests and two religious women, were severe
deprivation neurotics who had been incapacitated to various
degrees for many years. One had been diagnosed schizophrenic
and her condition had steadily worsened over the years while
receiving excessive doses of tranquilizers. One had been diagnosed correctly as a manic depressive, but like many persons
with this diagnosis had all the symptoms of a deprivation neurotic. He was treated as such while on lithium, and in psychotherapy and daily living learned new ways which proved increasingly rewarding in terms of leading a healthy, independent
life. The other two had been treated elsewhere (on more than
one occasion) symptomatically for their depression and psychosomatic disorders.

The advantages of this living-in arrangement which for some
lasted as long as twelve months were several. First, those of a
consistently affirming atmosphere unaffected by clinical con-
cepts and theories or utilitarian motivations, and generated by
a truly Christian way of life and respect for all living beings.
Second, those of being able to deal almost instantly and "on the
spot" with psychopathology. Although all four were most considerate in trying not to be a burden to the members of their
therapist's family they could not always hide their feelings of
depression or irritation. As far as the family was concerned this
never was met by any criticism or rejection, but accepted as a
normal part of life. Thus they were affirmed in the most undeveloped aspect of their beings, their emotional lives. Since the
patients could not hide from those who irritated them, as is
possible in any conventional treatment setting with a larger
number of patients, they were forced to confront each other
either in the twice-weekly group therapy sessions or in their
living and recreational quarters. Thus their immature ways of
relating were more quickly exposed and new, healthier ways
were taught explicitly in individual and group therapy, but also
implicitly by observation and imitation of the ways the parents

and their children related to one another. All expressed at various times their amazement at how the children were allowed to display their emotions freely, and received corrective criticism or comment only when the display was unreasonable or inappropriate. In general it can be said that therapy was more effective because of the intensity of emotional involvements, the frequency of daily encounters, both formal and informal, with the therapist, and the consistently affirming atmosphere created by the totally involved members of the family.

Because it is impossible to enumerate here all the other interesting aspects of this "reverse family therapy" we want to limit ourselves to the following two comments. This type of community living can never be therapeutic, nor should it ever be attempted, unless the adult members of the family possess a high degree, and the children an adequate degree relative to their age, of unselfish love of others. It is under circumstances such as these that it becomes fully evident that *affirmation therapy is not a method* or a way of *doing* things. Affirmation is purely a way of *being* that cannot be pretended, but has to be authentic if it is to be fruitful. Obviously, the members of the family could never pretend such affirmation for a prolonged period of time, nor bear up cheerfully under the occasional stressful atmosphere.

By the same token, we do not advise anyone to undertake a similar arrangement unless the home provides sufficient space to protect each person's privacy and adequate opportunity to be by oneself even for recreation. We were fortunate in this "experiment" to have in addition to eight bedrooms a large recreation room on the third floor of an old colonial house, and both front and rear staircases leading to the top floor. This provided ample opportunity for each resident to come and go without inconvenience to the others.[6]

1—The same desire has also been expressed in a different manner. It was described by a woman patient in a letter to us: "At times I make myself as small as possible; I pull my knees under my chin and crawl into the corner of an armchair. Then I take a large bowl of warm milk in both my hands, and sip it slowly. When I do this, I feel as if I was drinking from my mother's breast."

2—The Picture Section of the *Minneapolis Sunday Tribune* of April 3, 1966, carried a photograph of two college freshmen girls surrounded by a "landslide of cuddly creatures" under the heading "Why Teddy Bears Go to College." The psychology professor at the college attended by these two freshmen advised parents to send their daughters' teddy bears along, since "stuffed animals help girls bridge the gap between home and campus." From his surveys at two other universities he had found that more than 80 percent of the 1200 co-eds interviewed had three or more inanimate creatures in their room, while 40 percent of the male students also owned stuffed animals. The co-eds gave as their reasons for keeping stuffed animals in their room, "They keep me from getting homesick," "They cheer me up," "They keep me company," or "They give me someone to talk to." The male students stated most of their stuffed animals had been gifts from girl friends and were kept in cars instead of rooms. The psychology professor arrived at the conclusion that "stuffed animals, like books and ball games, are an integral part of college life." In our opinion, the professor would have drawn somewhat more profound conclusions if he had been familiar with the syndrome of deprivation neurosis and with unaffirmed individuals.

3—Not long ago we read in a newspaper about an irate woman who entered the office of a bishop with her husband, an ex-priest, and exclaimed, "Here, you can have this back. I thought I married a man two years ago, but he proved to be nothing more than a boy!"

4—In our opinion, the reason why such an alarming number of ordained priests and professed religious have defected in recent decades must be sought more in the factor of non-affirmation than in connection with repressed sexual needs. The same factor seems to play a significant role in the readiness of so many Catholics for ecumenical amalgamation, even at the price of doctrinal compromise. This strongly suggests the need for an affirmed hierarchy capable of affirming others.

5—A set of three tape cassettes entitled *Affirmation and Psychic Incarnation for Emotionally and Spiritually Troubled Persons* is commercially available to facilitate the process of emotional growth and integration. For information on the use and cost of this set, send long, self-addressed, stamped envelope to its author, C. W. Baars, M.D., 326 Highview Dr., San Antonio, Texas 78228.

6—We consider it necessary to draw the reader's attention to the fact that not every treatment or counseling center, nor every psychiatrist or psychologist claiming to provide affirmation therapy, can be assumed to practice this therapy correctly as described in this book. Frequently investigation of such claims will reveal little more than a form of self-affirmation or assertive training and some probing type of psychotherapy. The full description of the deprivation neurosis originated with its discoverer, Anna A. Terruwe, M.D. The same is true for the use of the terms *affirmation, self-affirmation, non-affirmation* and *pseudo-affirmation* in connection with emotional illness. Persons making contrary claims are either confusing the maternal deprivation syndrome with the syndrome of the deprivation neurosis, or have failed to make a thorough study of the world psychiatric literature. The original description of the deprivation or frustration neurosis may be found in *The Neurosis in the Light of Rational Psychology* by A.A.A. Terruwe, M.D., translated by C. W. Baars, M. D., P. J. Kenedy & Sons, New York, 1960, and in *De Frustratie Neurose* by Dr. A. A. A. Terruwe, J. J. Romen & Zonen, Roermond en Maaseik, 1962.

# CHAPTER VIII

# PERSONAL HISTORIES OF SOME DEPRIVATION NEUROTICS

## 1. *Paranoid Delusions and Behavior*

A thirty-five-year-old Catholic priest came to us in the company of his religious superior, who provided the following history. During the preceding several months the priest's behavior in the cloister had shown remarkable and unusual changes. He preferred to be alone in his room, refused to join the other members of his community for meals or spiritual exercises, and when he had to go to another part of the cloister or leave the building, he kept looking around in a furtive manner. Not long before he had told his superior that people were plotting against him, that newspaper and magazine articles referred to him, and that drivers were tooting their horns in a special way when they passed the cloister. He had insisted that the cloister's telephone switchboard and its operator be investigated, as he was certain that somebody was listening in on all his calls. He repeatedly accused himself of being guilty of compromising the reputation of the community as well as that of the priesthood.

Until this rather sudden change in personality, the patient had been a most friendly and helpful man, liked by everyone he met. He had performed his priestly duties exceedingly well, was an excellent speaker, and always attracted people by his sympathetic understanding of their personal difficulties. His superior further told us that the patient was the second son in a family of five children, and that as far as he knew, the family had no history of insanity, alcoholism, or degenerative disease. Aside from a lack of emotional rapport between the members of the family, which was also socially isolated, there had been no serious difficulties at home. The patient had received most of his education in a religious boarding school and had done better than average in his studies for the priesthood. Everybody had the greatest expectations for his future. As far as the superior knew, the patient had always enjoyed good physical health.

At the time of our first examination of the patient, he impressed us as being extremely fearful, although he reacted appropriately and spoke freely about his delusions. He did this, however, in a whisper, after requesting that the window of the examining room be closed and inquiring about the possible presence of hidden recording devices in the room. He had but one desire, namely, to be put away in a hospital, because he felt that in that way he would be safe from being taken into custody by the police authorities.

He showed a tremor of the hands, which were clammy; his pupils were dilated and unsteady; his muscle stretch reflexes were markedly increased, with extension of the reflexogenic areas. Body hair distribution was normal, as were secondary sex characteristics. Routine laboratory tests, including glucose tolerance test and spinal fluid examination, were all within normal limits. These tests were done in the hospital to which he was admitted immediately following our initial interview. Temperature and pulse curves were normal, showing normal day and night fluctuations. The patient had no trouble falling asleep; he slept all through the night and was not bothered by early morning awakening.

We considered the following three differential diagnoses: sensitive paranoia of Kretschmer; early organic brain syndrome with psychosis; and deprivation neurosis. We were inclined to favor the last diagnosis because we had observed similar paranoid ideas develop in other deprivation neurotics when they had failed seriously, either objectively or subjectively, in their duties and obligations. Another factor that favored this diagnosis was the patient's excellent rapport with others. To be as certain as possible of the diagnosis, especially in view of the therapeutic approach to be decided upon, we requested specialized psychometric testing. The Rorschach findings made it possible to exclude with a very high degree of certainty the existence of an organic psychosis, while the characteristic features of deprivation neurosis could be clearly demonstrated in the test results.

Following these preliminary investigations, we instituted *insulin subcoma treatment*. After three weeks the patient's general physical condition had much improved. As far as his mental condition was concerned, his delusions of reference involving his immediate surroundings had disappeared; the curtains and windows were allowed to be open; his joking remarks about his earlier ideas that the nurses were spying on him showed that he was developing some insight into his illness. The most promising positive result, however, was the marked degree of confidence he developed in his psychiatrist during these three weeks. Another favorable prognostic omen at this early stage in therapy was his ability to accept the psychiatrist's ideas concerning his delusions without finding it necessary to justify or explain them himself.

In the fourth week, while the patient continued with his rest cure in the hospital, we initiated more extensive discussions. He confirmed the rather limited history given to us by his superior and added considerable detail. He indicated that his fearful paranoid state had been brought on soon after he became aware of feelings of tenderness toward a ten-year-old boy. Nothing objectively reprehensible had occurred and whatever contact there had been between them would never have been considered out of the ordinary by any normally developed man. Yet, this patient interpreted his relationship with the boy as unequivocal evidence of homosexuality, something about which the patient had worried for years.

His psychosexual development appeared to have taken a normal course. His first nocturnal emissions had occurred when he was fourteen. As he had received intelligent and sound sex education, it was not surprising that he had never developed neurotic fears of sexual matters in general. He never masturbated. It appeared, however, that on a strictly psychological level he had never experienced feelings of love, except for children. In our discussions it became clear to him that there had never been any emotional ties between himself and his parents, brothers, and sisters. Expressions of love and tenderness between the members of his family had been practically non-existent, and although in his youth he had never consciously felt the need for such expressions, it was now, in retrospect, evident to him that they had been lacking. Never in his adolescent years had there been anything to suggest erotic feelings toward girls, or any desire for dating and social intercourse.

These discoveries on the part of the patient led us to a discussion of the *meaning of tenderness* in the emotional life of man in general, and of the child in particular. We explained to him that tenderness represents a beautiful expression of man's emotional life and is prompted by his deep-seated need for love—for giving as well as receiving love. While this tenderness is required in every child for the affirmation of its being, it is greater when the child's emotional life is more sensitive. In view of the fact that our patient had never found this tenderness at home, it was quite understandable that this need emerged at a time when, in his work as a teacher in a preparatory seminary, it could be so easily directed to young boys. We further explained that this was not at all an indication of being a homosexual, but only a manifestation of a human need frustrated in a certain developmental phase of his emotional life, and that it would disappear by itself once the gradual growing process had been successfully resumed. That his need for tenderness was so intense stemmed from the fact that he possessed a basically sensitive nature. He had artistic talent and composed many poems which in this stage of his life dealt chiefly with the beauty of nature, which he was capable of experiencing without fear. It was obvious that the patient had little difficulty in acquiring a thorough understanding of the things we were discussing and not long after he began to experience a sense of liberation resulting from his newly gained insights.

After nine weeks of hospitalization he was well enough to continue with treatment as an outpatient. It soon appeared, however, that his delusions of reference concerning his former community had far from disappeared. Fortunately, it was possible to maintain the degree of improvement obtained so far by transferring him to a different milieu. In view of his scientific interests, we advised him to begin working on a thesis.

In the ensuing weeks his delusions detached themselves more and more from the difficulties of everyday life, so that we were able to gain a better understanding of his more fundamental psychological difficulties. In essence, these appeared to revolve around two basic factors, namely, a deeply rooted feeling of guilt, and a need to acquiesce to others in every respect.

His feeling of guilt appeared to derive from his conviction that he was inadequate in everything. This was not difficult to see, because his emotional life had evidently not developed beyond an infantile stage, so that, being a priest, he was obliged to live far beyond his psychological capacities. His compulsive need to acquiesce manifested itself in exaggerated friendliness and politeness. He never dared to make his own wishes known, much less to satisfy them. By the same token he kept his opinions to himself if there was a chance they might offend others.

As it was important for his recovery for him to become aware of these factors and understand the reasons for their existence, we discussed them in reference to numerous events in his past life. We showed him that his feelings of guilt were rooted in an actual failure to respond emotionally to others, which was in no way the fault of his free will, or something he could change himself. It was, we told him, something which he had to accept for the time being, until he had made further progress in his psychological development, when it would disappear by itself. We warned him specifically against any deliberate attempts on his part to compensate for this shortcoming in his emotional life.

His seemingly excessive friendliness stemmed from his need to receive friendly recognition from others. This, however, would lead to conflict and frustration in the patient when somebody treated him unkindly in act or words or looks, or even when the patient only imagined that somebody had been unkind. Under those circumstances he would react as all deprivation neurotics do—by being kind and taking heed not to displease the other person. Our treatment consisted of showing him how this *subservient attitude* could bring on only a feeling of displeasure, because it was actually an irrational act. In other words, one unpleasant feeling (the one caused by the other person's unkindness) was merely displaced by another, more pathological, unpleasant feeling. We explained that the only proper attitude is to recognize the other's unkindness for what it is—an ill-mannered act—and endure it calmly as such. Such a reaction not only restores the "hurt" feeling, but it gives the patient an opportunity to show that he accepts the other for what he is.

In the meantime an intense emotional rapport with the therapist developed in the patient. He told us that save for the young boy mentioned before, we were the only one who meant anything to him. This attitude was well illustrated in a letter which he once wrote us, which opened with the words "Dear Mother" and was signed "Your child." We took this opportunity to discuss with him the fact that every human contact, in order to endure, must be based on the *actual objective relationship* between the human beings involved. In our case the relationship was that of an adult man, a priest, and his physician. It was certainly true that within this relationship there existed an even closer tie resulting from the fact that his physician's affirmation of him caused his psychic life to unfold, precisely as happens when a mother and her child have a healthy positive relationship. However, although this was a very special, real, and personal relationship, it did not follow that it should distort the factual relationship upon which it was based. The patient, an intelligent man desirous of knowing the truth, was much relieved by this newly gained insight which provided him with the necessary understanding to handle his emotional experience in a positive manner that promised well for the future. Except for physical contact, he experienced every measure of confidence and surrender with his therapist that a child experiences with its mother. His need for reassurance was typically illustrated, for example, by his many lengthy letters in which he shared with us his day-to-day experiences. This is a characteristic need of practically all deprivation neurotics, for they are basically uncertain of themselves and they gain strength from the fact that the person who has their confidence knows everything they do and affirms them. We, therefore, calmly left things as they were: when the patient became more mature emotionally, his letter writing became less frequent and finally stopped altogether.

When, during the course of therapy, the patient developed an increasing need to play—he himself called it a waste of time to play games—we explained that in his stage of mental development his sensory faculties were not yet capable of directing themselves in an orderly manner at any given object. Any given faculty can do this only after it has fully matured. Therefore, it would be much more fitting for him to apply himself to practicing the functions of his various faculties and thus experience what Karl Buhler calls the *Funktionslust*—the pleasure of exercising one's natural faculties—and what Aquinas describes as the natural delight which follows upon the normal exercise of a faculty. Following our advice, he tried to be as uninhibited as possible—within reasonable limits, of course—in his desire to play. It was not long thereafter that his nephews and nieces promoted him to the nicest uncle of the family, because he participated so pleasantly in their games. The patient emphasized the fact that it was not he who played with the children, but they with him, and that he experienced the excitement of their games precisely as children do. He would become angry when he was the loser and it was a real effort for him not to show this. He told us also that there was nothing that absorbed him and held his attention as much as these games. To enable him to take full advantage of developing these feelings further, we advised him to go swimming often and to take daily exercises with a physical therapist.

In the months that followed, he developed various interests that he had never known in his younger years. He became an ardent photographer and an enthusiastic spectator at soccer games. Such typical spectator games as soccer and basketball provide adults with a socially approved outlet for their *Funktionslust*, for here people from all walks of life can shout, stamp their feet, and jump up and down as much as they please.

This change in personality development also affected the patient's writing of his thesis, which we had recommended earlier in the treatment. He had found it became increasingly more difficult to apply himself to this task, because he was too distracted to study regularly. He had actually never been able to do so, not even in his school and college years, and he had always blamed it on laziness. It had only been because of his superior intelligence that he had been able to complete his studies with a minimum of effort. But now he realized that he ought to study in the same manner that a child plays, that is, for the pleasure of doing it rather than solely to obtain a certain goal.

There is a third aspect of the therapy of deprivation neurosis which, like the matter of reassuring the patient of his innate worth and enabling him to experience the *Funktionslust*, may present problems for solution. This is the necessary development of a patient's feeling of love. Without the actual experience of tactile tenderness, this feeling cannot sufficiently develop. In this patient the need for tenderness had already been directed to young boys. Now it was impossible for him to continue his relationship with the young boy for whom he had such feelings of tenderness, although objectively their relationship had been most proper and there was no danger that this honest man would abuse it. It so happened, however, that the patient had an opportunity to teach in another country where the display of affection between adults and children is less inhibited. During his year in that country he had ample occasion to receive and give tactile tendernesses, which, of course, was at all times free of any sexual connotation. He sensed that he was becoming more mature in those months, and this also became evident from the content of the poems that he sent us from time to time, and from the fact that he had less need to share with us all the events of his everyday life. He gradually developed emotional rapport with adults, and to his great surprise he noticed that people began to consider him witty and popular. His attraction for boys decreased more and more and finally disappeared altogether. Instead he developed a normal interest in women and girls, with which he was able to cope without any difficulty.

Five years after the beginning of therapy our patient's phenotype had changed to the point of being unrecognizable; he had become a normal adult man. His delusions had disappeared early in the course of treatment as a result of his affirmative rapport with the therapist; the same was true of the feelings of guilt on which these delusions were based. He had become independent in his relationship with others and it no longer even occurred to him to try to please others constantly. He spoke his mind freely and led his own life in an independent though, of course, considerate manner.

## 2. *Psychic Incarnation in Therapy*

This case history offers, we believe, a further excellent illustration of deprivation neurosis as it has been described in the pages of this book. It is a remarkable case history for two reasons: First, because of the unusually consistent manner in which the patient applied her newly gained insights to her condition; and second, because of the steady and systematic progress of her recovery.

When the patient first came to us for help, she was twenty-nine years old, the oldest of six children from a family of good social standing. Her life at home had been difficult, as her mother was probably also a deprivation neurotic. The patient had never received any tenderness from her, nor had she ever been affirmed by her in her way of life and behavior. No matter what she did, it had always been wrong and her mother had always corrected her in everything. Nevertheless, her mother had not hesitated to seek consolation and help for her own marital difficulties by telling the patient, ever since she was six years old, about all her intimate problems with her husband. And as far as her father was concerned, he too had never given his daughter any positive affirmation of her being.

The girl was of superior intelligence, and after finishing school, she studied pharmacology. At the time of her first interview she was employed as an assistant pharmacist. Her physical condition was excellent, and she was free of physical complaints.

Her reason for seeking help was her inability to go on living. Lacking every bit of emotional rapport with others, she had to will herself to be friendly in all her social and occupational contacts. It was this effort which had become virtually impossible for her, and she was afraid that her condition would become intolerable.

At first we saw her at irregular intervals, but much less frequently than was necessary and desirable because of the great distance between her hometown and ours. In order for her to have somebody to talk to during the weeks between her interviews, we referred her to an understanding priest in her hometown. Shortly thereafter, on Mother's Day, she made a serious attempt at suicide because, she told us later, she interpreted this referral as an indication that we wanted to get rid of her and she intended, at least unconsciously, to show us that she needed us and not the priest. As a result of this suicidal attempt, she was admitted to a hospital and during her stay there arrangements were made for her to see us on a weekly basis. This was the real beginning of therapy.

The first remarkable development was her insistence on a complete break with her former life. It was here that we became aware of her previously mentioned character trait, namely, that she was unbelievably logical in doing what she considered right. She did this down to the smallest detail, without ever making allowances for any of the consequences. She broke her relationship with her parents and family, as all this was part of her earlier life which she detested thoroughly. She did not even want to talk about her parents anymore. If she had to refer to them for some reason, she did not use the words "father" or "mother" but employed substitute words which were free of any emotional connotation.

Even the things she possessed had to go: her clothes, her books, and her furniture. She wanted to have nothing that would bring up memories of the past. Her whole life had to begin anew, and moreover it had to begin again through us and with us. It had to be developed in complete dependence on us. As far as she was concerned, we had given her this new life which she wanted to experience in everything without exception.

She did not want to do anything without us. Even the clothes she wanted to purchase had to be seen by us first. Everything was brought to our office—located in our residence—even if this meant the trouble of bringing a suitcase. She would not use any article until we had seen it, not even if she had an urgent need for it. She made photographs of her room so that we could see that also; only then did it become hers. The same was true for her closets and drawers, so that we could see where and how she put all her belongings.

We also had to teach her how to take care of her appearance, because when she first came to us for help she neglected herself completely. Only when she came to see us would she make a slight effort to look presentable. We had to persuade her to take a bath regularly, to wash her hair, and to groom her hands and nails.

It was difficult for her to get up in the morning in time to take care of her nails. But when she was allowed to give an accounting of this task to us, it was no longer difficult. It was her own idea to draw a little doll on the calendar for each day of the month that she had cleaned her nails. These drawings she brought along at each interview and it was then our task to inspect and approve every one of them. During our vacations she would neglect herself again, at least during the early part of therapy, because at those times we were not there to give approval.

In the beginning she did not care for clothes at all. She was indifferent about her looks. When she was in need of a new dress, she would order one on approval and bring it along on her next visit, put it on in the office for us to see, and, if we approved of it, she would buy it. Gradually she developed more interest and began to take care of matters of dress herself. At present she is a well-groomed and elegantly dressed young lady.

We also had to teach her all kinds of household tasks such as sewing, crocheting, knitting, darning. She had never wanted to learn those things in earlier years and had even refused outright to try her hand at them, because she had always seen her mother doing these things and, therefore, did not want any part of them. But after we had taught her these activities, she enjoyed them fully.

These were the changes in her exterior life. Those in her emotional life became evident soon after the start of therapy. At first she did not want to accept her bodily existence because she had not been born from us. To this we replied that her psychic being was more important than her physical being, and that she could receive the former from us. This insight satisfied her and she began at once to grow and to live through the various phases of development. She often expressed in drawings the way she felt. They made it abundantly clear that she felt completely like a little child.

When she had grown older emotionally, she preferred to sit on the floor at our feet. It is remarkable how many deprivation neurotic patients prefer this to sitting on a chair. Somehow the chair seems to disturb the psychomotor reactions of a growing person.

The growth of man's emotional life is being manifested in the feeling of security he experiences in being with another person. Man has to step outside of himself and direct himself toward another being. This takes place first in symbols, and afterwards in reality. So it happened with this patient.

One day she asked us for a teddy bear. The teddy bear, the bunny, and other toy animals are a symbol of "the other," albeit a symbol which one can manipulate as much as one wants without the risk of resistance or rebellion. With them, it is safe to become what one potentially is.

The patient got her teddy bear and began to develop toward it all kinds of feelings: love, tenderness, care, to name only a few. The teddy bear got the name of "Winnie," and accompanied her on all her visits to us, for she wanted it to share in everything.

Later on the patient developed a desire for a doll. This was a step forward, for a doll represents more than an animal, namely, a human being. The little doll "Robinet" got a place next to Winnie and shared in all his experiences.

Her emotional rapport with other people first developed through us in regard to those she knew played a role in our personal life. Of course, such contact was never actually made, as the physician-patient relationship ordinarily must exclude the patient from the physician's private life. The patient always respected this fully. It was only in her imagination that our parental home began to play a most sympathetic role.

Real contacts then followed. First with the children in the street where she lived. Interestingly enough, these contacts were only negative in the beginning; she stuck out her tongue at the children and quarrelled with them. But later her feelings began to change and she became friendly with all the neighborhood children.

Time went on and these contacts were gradually extended to adults until at present she has, without any effort on her part, a normal emotional rapport with her fellow human beings. This rapport no longer is willed; it is simply determined by her feelings. The only difficult rapport is still that which she has with the members of her family, but there are indications that this too is improving.

This whole process of emotional evolution progressed in a regular fashion, except that during our vacations she often disintegrated and as a result quarrelled with everybody. During these periods she was without her main source of support and unsure of herself. At the time of this writing this no longer happens since her emotional growth is virtually complete.

Mention should be made of the fact that from the time she began therapy, she was able to maintain her composure toward the outside world. Weekly sessions gave her an opportunity to discuss the many difficulties which made themselves felt repeatedly, and gave her sufficient inner calm to carry on outwardly. She did her work and kept up with her studies in order to make progress in her profession.

A final word, concerning her *religious growth*. When she first came to us she had, as far as her feelings were concerned, broken completely with her religion. She never attended church and did not pray, since for her God was merely a robot who imposed his coercion on people, as she expressed it. She felt that we had saved her from the terror of her religion. We accepted all this calmly, of course, and did not make any attempt to change her attitude. Very gradually, this anti-religious attitude disappeared by itself to make room again in her heart for the faith and the love of Christ. All this, too, was clearly portrayed in the drawings she made during her years of therapy. Some of these drawings were accompanied by accounts of her religious feelings in early life, and as they underwent a gradual transformation in therapy. A few of them are reproduced here.

\*     \*     \*     \*     \*     \*

I am at Doctor's.
Doctor takes me in her arms to take a glimpse at the past. This can be done only together with Doctor. Otherwise the past drags you back again, don't you see?
In the past I was in a Church, and one of her churches was the . . . church in Amsterdam. It was so big.

And cold and gloomy. There were many people, almost
always, who stared at you and thought immediately
all kinds of things of you; it divided you in a thousand-
million fragments of what they thought, and not a
piece of me was left intact. But Doctor has claimed
every bit of them and assembled and taken me along with
Her—what a blessing! When you entered that church, you
had to make your way through all their glances, and
when you sat in a pew, their glances pierced and
penetrated through our coat. Even if they did not know
a thing about you they would think and divide you
up into bad qualities. Going to church was horrible
because you always met people—enemies, all of them.
In the Church and her churches there are billions of
possibilities of sin, small ones, big ones and mortal sins;
before you know it, you have fallen into the latter even
before your First Holy Communion. That Mary of
them towers above everything; she has the time of her
life on feastdays and especially with Christmas, when
she speculates on the feelings of those people of the
church by acting as a so-called "mother." The Church
also preaches that she is the paragon of sacrifice; besides
there is nothing of which she is not the paragon,
according to them. When you have know-how of
everything and most of all of her, plus the Church it is
very difficult to escape from their sphere of influence
and their grip.

*    *    *    *    *    *

*God creates the world.*

God is a robot.
He is inherent in the intellectual products of his brain.
Beneath the roof of his skull lies the nucleus
of his existence in the form of the Trinity.

Because he lives exclusively from his intellect he is an
unapproachable, ice cold, calculating individual.
He exists therefore only partly
And not in the fullness of the living like Doctor.
He thinks exclusively in formulas and
his church calls that "logic."
But what is logic without Love.
Like the cadaver of Mister X of which one
would swear that it is Mister X.
But Doctor is wise and loving and logical.
Therefore Doctor is Her Logic vibrantly alive,
The Logic of God and his church is therefore
suffocating. They possess no Love,
They are like machines, one cannot live in their world.
Doctor contains Earth and Heaven.

*     *     *     *     *     *

*The shepherd who lost his way.*

After hearing the Message of the Angel, he and the other
shepherds had set out on their way. But as he had to
think out many things he did not notice that he drifted
away from the others.

Now he had to go on alone and he does not know
exactly to where for the star has accompanied the
other shepherds. But arrive at his destination he will,
for he will search and search until he finds Christ.

He has not made much headway yet for when he
turns around he can still see the stable and his sheep.

He has a very special and beautiful gift for Christ.
He holds it up high in his hands, very carefully, so
nothing will happen to it, for he is quite sure that he still
has a long way to go. Nobody is around on the long
and lonely road, and there are thunder clouds in the sky.
But he belongs to Doctor, doesn't he, and therefore
everything is well.

\*   \*   \*   \*   \*   \*

Doctor, you are to me all in one father and venerable mother; you are my secure home where I may live here on earth as well as later when we shall be together with Christ.

Doctor's glowing Love transcends life-choking ties. Like the strong woman of the Gospel she cuts, through the miracle of her Love, the umbilical cord which only artificially supported the exterior life.

Nevertheless, in her understanding Love, she sees to it that together with her the child, to whom she gives birth in the loving reception of her heart, respects the good of the two custodians whose task to put life into the child she assumed. For those two gave of their talents to the extent of their capacities.

Thus the Doctor provides the vital spark of consolation for those who remained behind and for the child in her heart to whom she reveals the miracle of its existence; the miracle of being at once large and small. She teaches the child the first words of Love and joy. She teaches it to walk and hold its hand in times of light and darkness, of rebellion and surrender, of deep-felt joy and sadness.

The child is still on its way. But no matter at what moment of its travel it looks up, whether by day or at night, she sees the Doctor. As her Love encompasses Heaven and Earth (even beyond the borders of this life) everything becomes one immense exuberant adventure.

Doctor gives me the joy of her Love.

\*   \*   \*   \*   \*   \*

\*   \*   \*   \*   \*   \*

### 3. *Playing in a Sandbox*

In spite of his size, six feet, four inches and 230 pounds, the thirty-five-year-old high school teacher was not at all impressive when he entered our office and in the armchair assumed and maintained for an entire hour a posture characteristic of his feelings of inferiority and utter worthlessness. Hunched forward with his head between his shoulders, elbows bent at his sides, and his hands and forearms folded in front of his chest, he reminded one of the fetal position. All during the hour he stared continuously at the floor, spoke haltingly and with a pronounced stammer. We had been advised that he had been diagnosed a chronic ambulatory schizophrenic, and had been given a total of forty-six deep insulin coma treatments in the past year, but without noticeable improvement. The patient had been discharged after a year of therapy with a hopeless prognosis.

Although he had some of the clinical features of catatonic schizophrenia, it was not hard to make the proper diagnosis in view of our immediate rapport, his feeling of loneliness and deep depression, his fear and distrust of people in general, his utter lack of self-confidence and constant self-debasement, his avowed need to avoid criticism, and his attempts to receive recognition and acceptance by going out of his way to please others, whether by hard work or giving into their demands and arguments. He had quit teaching two years before as he could not maintain proper discipline and felt ill at ease with the other faculty members. The only contacts he cared for were younger people who were kind to him.

His background was typical of all patients with deprivation neurosis. His mother was cold and unloving, and always ready with ridicule, scoldings, and punishments for any conduct that caused her the slightest inconvenience, such as leaving dirty clothes on the floor or coming in with muddy shoes, or for behavior which was considered a threat to her authority or was not in conformity with the standards and expectations, real or assumed, of the neighbors. His father was so quiet and passive,

so submissive and undemonstrative, that none of his seven children ever got to know him, or knew whether they meant anything to him. But outside the home he apparently meant something to others, for at his death more than two hundred persons
had Masses said for the repose of his soul! All this, of course,
the patient did not tell us until much later in therapy, when he
had come to trust us fully without reservations or fear.

So great was the patient's need to be loved and his fear of
being rejected, that he used to allow his younger brother to win
in competitive sports at every opportunity: "I want to tell you
something, Doctor; I was much better than my brother, but I
always let him win! . . . I've never been loved by anybody,
Doctor; I was always told I was no good."

Early in therapy he was advised to cut down on his working
hours as a maintenance man and to do his assigned work at a
slower and more relaxed pace. He was advised to take a break
as soon as he started to perspire or become tired. This he found
difficult to do at first, as he was always afraid of incurring the
displeasure or wrath of his superiors, who often took advantage
of his too agreeable demeanor by assigning him too many tasks.
He had little difficulty in understanding the nature of his emotional illness, and saw the importance of daring to cut down on
his excessive energy, which he employed solely to counteract
his overwhelming fear of his environment. He realized that only
in this way could there be created a more relaxed inner atmosphere and attitude in which his undeveloped pleasure emotions
could begin to grow slowly.

Four months after the start of our weekly sessions he told us
how he liked to daydream about trucks, and loved to sit at the
side of the road watching them go by. And when he had a
chance to talk to a truck driver—the very people his mother had
considered the lowliest of all men—he felt the happiest. Because
we affirmed him in these desires and encouraged him to find
even more time to sit and watch the trucks go by, it was not
long before he dared to confide—although not without much
embarrassment—that his greatest desire was to play in a sandbox,

and also with toys, both things he had never been allowed to do as a child. We suggested that it might be a good idea if he were to get himself some toy trucks and other toys to play with in the privacy of his room, and to keep his eyes open for any opportunity to play in the sand without danger of being embarrassed by others. On his next visit he reported happily that he was finding much joy in playing for hours with his toy trucks every night before going to bed. A little later he told us how he enjoyed reading *Teenage Tales* and other stories for children and young people, and how he liked listening to music and on occasion found himself singing along with the artist. He also began to feel more relaxed in his work on the maintenance crew since his fellow-workers were straightforward, uncomplicated people who treated him as a human being, and often prompted him not to kill himself in his job, especially since his hard working made them look bad in the eyes of their boss.

The intensity of his twisted emotional life was well demonstrated one day when he told us how he had waved at the engineer of a passing train and how happy he had been when the engineer had tooted in return. But then he asked immediately, "Did I do wrong, Doctor? Why did the engineer toot back?" We reassured him that he had done well by his spontaneous display of friendliness and that the engineer must have liked him for waving at him.

When he told us that he had always wanted to play cards but had never done so for fear of making mistakes, we taught him to play cribbage, a game he had been especially desirous of learning. It was soon obvious, when he had caught on to the rules of the game and played it well enough, that he avoided winning. When we let him win his first game in spite of his efforts to lose, it was evident that he felt most uncomfortable. Asked whether anything was wrong he replied that he was not happy at all for having won and that he was afraid that we would not like him any more as a result of his having caused us to lose the game. After a discussion of the irrationality of allowing oneself to be dominated in everything, even a friendly card game, by the fear of being disliked and thus feeding and multiplying his fears unnecessarily, he really enjoyed winning his second game of cribbage on the next visit. Several times during these card playing sessions he remarked, "Whenever I shuffle the cards I have a hard time stopping—it is as if I cannot let go of the cards."

That the feeling of being no good, of always being in the wrong, and of having done wrong and thus deserving the wrath of others is often intense and deep-seated in deprivation neurotics was revealed one day. He once told how a friend had taken him for a ride in his car the previous weekend. The patient had noticed another car following them for two or three blocks, and became intensely afraid that someone was after him for doing something wrong.

Approximately ten months after the start of therapy the patient was assigned by his employer to a new job in a more remote location and with different co-workers. Like all deprivation neurotics he feared this change, for it meant meeting and living with new people under difficult circumstances and regulations. For deprivation neurotics such a move, rather than providing a chance of making new friends, is the cause of the exhausting task of discovering what new people are like, learning what they think and feel in order to know how best to please them and avoid becoming the victim of their dislike or anger. Thus, new encounters constitute a veritable effort for deprivation neurotics; in their minds such encounters are fraught with danger and full of the risk of making mistakes. The first impulse is to resist change of any consequence and much encouragement is required to overcome this fear.

In this particular case, the change of job and environment proved to be fortunate for the patient. The more distant assignment happened to be near a river with a sandy beach, while the surrounding forest provided seclusion and privacy for the realization of his fondest wish "to play in the sand like a carefree child." Not wanting to wait until the next visit to tell the good news, he wrote us, "Doctor, I think the most fun is playing in the river, which is very low at some points. I love to crawl and run through the water and play in the sand. But the best thing is down on all fours in the mud and going right along—plus playing in the sand. Why is it, Doctor, that I feel so good lying in the sand?" We assured him that it was good for him to experience such pleasant things as water and sand, pointing out that the more he dared to enjoy them without feeling guilty the more he would grow emotionally.[1]

That same summer he went fishing for the first time in his life. When his first catch turned out to be a big one, he had someone take a picture of himself and his prize catch, and proudly brought it along on his next visit. But it was not the usual picture of a man holding a fish which is dangling from the hook in its mouth. Instead it showed the patient happily and tenderly looking at his fish—cradled safely in the crook of his arm!

His emotional life grew noticeably during those months of playing in the river and the sand, especially when he was able to share this fun for several weeks with a boy who was visiting relatives in the neighborhood. They splashed water at one another, played ball, and did all the things young boys do in the summer months. He became obviously much less tense during our visits and allowed his arms to rest on the arms of the chair in a more relaxed manner. He looked at us more frequently and his conversation became more animated and outspoken. In view of the fact that he had become more aware of his feelings, he also began to worry about what he might do if he allowed himself to become angry. We repeatedly encouraged him to accept his angry feelings and not repress them out of fear that they could lead to words or actions which might displease others. We advised him to repeatedly reassure himself that it was all right to feel angry before attempting to express his anger or irritation, even if it were to take weeks or months before he would be ready to do so. If he were to ignore this advice and begin to express his anger prematurely he would retard his progress because such expressions of anger could only be effected by repressing his fear of anger. That, of course, is as unhealthy as the repression of the emotion of anger itself is. At times he got a feeling that he was going to have a temper tantrum, something he never had had as a child ("I would have been kicked in the mouth, Doctor!"). By letting him talk about all the people he hated, and repeatedly affirming his feelings of hate and anger as natural and necessary psycho-biological responses to evil, he gradually learned to repress them less and less. And as he allowed these feelings to be expressed in words from time to time, he discovered that they never led to physical outbursts even though we had avoided warning him against them. At the same time he discovered to his satisfaction that people started to treat him with more respect whenever his anger aroused him to assert himself with them. Although this pleased him, he would often ask us whether he had done right, or he would say, "I shouldn't have done that, Doctor."

Three years after the start of therapy he became active in a program of physical exercises such as wrestling, judo, swimming, and track, as a result of which his hitherto poor coordination improved considerably. He got a position as a physical education instructor at a high school, and although his stammer had not completely disappeared he had no difficulty disciplining even the problem kids. After two years in that position he took part in the traditional introduction of the staff members at the start of the school year and got more applause than any of the others.

He still continues to visit us from time to time at irregular intervals, for the environment in which he must live is a difficult one and retards his emotional growth. He suffers much from the lack of sensitivity of other people to his need for friendship and love, busy and preoccupied as they are with their own work and interests. He looks forward to the day when he can live and work with people who accept and love him for himself, not just because of what his work can contribute to the community, but in their unselfish concern for his personal welfare. Without continued help and encouragement it becomes easier for him to see the shortcomings of others, which hurt him so much, for what they are, rather than to interpret them as evidence of his own worthlessness and inferiority. Understood in that way he can tolerate and forgive those persons for being blind to his needs and yet, in the suffering resulting from their selfishness, continue to mature toward becoming a free and happy human being.

### 4. *Too Old to Be Healed?*

The last account of this chapter was written by a woman in her mid-sixties after one year of affirmation therapy for severe depression and serious doubts about God and her Catholic faith. She describes here in verse and prose her feelings, thoughts and experiences before, during and after treatment.

A talented, witty, erudite music teacher, she had seen numerous psychiatrists over the years to no avail. Only her strong feeling that everyone would be better off if she "just disappeared" had motivated her to seek professional help once more. She manifested and related all the typical characteristics of a severe deprivation neurotic. She was physically and mentally exhausted from life-long pleasing others, but never herself, and from suppressing her feelings of inferiority and inadequacy by doing her work to perfection, by never refusing any extra assignments or volunteering for whatever work she thought others wanted done. She was convinced that "she was too old to be healed."

Her "after treatment" comments stress the urgent need on the part of religious communities, and for that matter, families and other groups to de-fuse entrenched utilitarian philosophies and value systems, and to establish an atmosphere where everyone is allowed to *be* and as such to contribute to the group by being herself in freedom. This, of course, is another way of saying that there is a great need for mutual affirmation in the presumably well members in the communities and families of the patient. Too many relatives and members of a religious community assume that, because they have not received psychiatric care, they are mature and affirming persons. This, of course, is to be expected when one does not know what is meant by maturity and affirmation. We hope that this personal account of one of our patients will dispel this ignorance and suggest to many ways and means of enriching their own lives and the lives of those who "broke down" and had to find the needed affirmation elsewhere.

BEFORE TREATMENT

### Emptiness

This is one of those times
When no one speaks the language that I know.
This is one of those endless days
When I must smile and make believe and try to show
A peace and gentleness and joy
I cannot feel,
Lest I destroy
Another's peace or cause a wound
In someone's happiness
Which I can never hope to heal.
This is a day when I would love so much
To reach out
But my hands are bound;
I have no power to touch.
And in my soul there can be found
No single gift to give
Nor single good to do!
There must be some small growths of love
    and selflessness within.
Why is it so impossible for me
To send them through?

### Pretending

Play games
Show interest
And approve
Make lips and cheek bones smile.

Continue thus pretending
They'll trust you for a while.

Behind you then—the looking glass
Will show their posture-planning
Within their eyes
And in the clutching of their hands.
They will not reach you with their minds;
There'll be no friendly spanning.

These are charades:
(We act and seem to trust.)
No other can decode them.
Even the doubtful aims we had
In entering them
Must tend soon to erode them.

### Fear

I am afraid of everyone and everything,
And I am often doubtful as to what to do;
Or if I choose, my actions cause
A side effect of guilt. My view
Of what I'm doing makes me pause
And fear that my decision has been wrong
Or selfish, or unwise or futile in some way,
Why can I never say,
"This is my choice—my act!" and be so strong
That waves of fear will go without me back to sea;
A sea of dark confusion and despair.
Once I was rescued breathless from its drowning scare,
Now I am walking hesitantly on the shore
Lest it should also proffer danger
As it seems to scrape and claw
And try to suck me quicksand-deep.
Would it be easier to go to sleep

And let all fade in depths of sinking sand
Or waves that with such power pull and draw?
Both can enfold me, wrap me round in peace,
But if there is a life to follow
Even my succumbing would not bring release.

## Too Cowardly to Trust

A need remains—
A word, an incident,
A clearing thought,
An understanding,
The opening or the closing of a door
Before I can be free.
I seem to see
A light directing me,
And then before
I dare to follow it
I see it disappear
And there is once again a mist,
Opaque and unrevealing—never clear;
And yet at times sufficient
In its visibility
To tantalize me to make search again.
I am too cowardly to trust:
Always and ever I must be so sure
There really is a light.
Before I start to follow
Night melts into night
Because I miss
The moment of the midnight sun.
One who lives thus by choice
Or circumstance in this dark land
Must walk in trust,
Hand holding hand holding hand
And move the minute that the light appears

Brief glowing and so far.
All else may fail—directing word,
Or clarifying thought,
The choice of opening or closing proper doors.
There is no leading star,
There is no other way
Save trust
To move through fear.

### Winter in My Soul

I have refused to sing
And in these days I have renounced
All right to song;
Yet in my soul a strong
And straining melody
Pleads to break through,
But I can never sing
When other sounds
Are beating like a frenzied storm
Against my ears
Tumbling together to destroy
The harmony of memory.

I would recall
The cherished beauty of
The art song of my life,
But all is hollow toneless sound.
That which I loved and strove to live,
That which I treasured well enough to give
To little eager ones,
To older wiser ones than I
I dare not touch
Even to give to them again.
Were they to reach out now
Expecting me to bring them song

They would find nothing coming
To their hopeful listening ears.
That which I loved
Can now bring only tears.

Sounds in this night
Are sounds from which my soul in fright
Must run away
And I do fear this way
So marked with blight,
For it is winter in my soul
And One there was Who warned against
A winter flight.

## Fear, Guilt, Grief

I cannot tolerate the thoughts
Now gathered in my mind:
I am afraid:
I feel a guilt for actions that I cannot face,
Plans I have not laid.
Even though judgment tells me
I have done or not done as I must—
When others clamor,
What they shout has too great thrust
To be ignored.
I cannot stand it, Lord.
I have returned again into that place
Of cold estrangement
And I find no trace
Of trust, or understanding or forgiveness
Or what they now proclaim
As reconciliation.
I stand here bearing blame
For what I find impossible for me
To carry through,

Let some strong person take my place
For there is nothing I can do.
And now the ultimate in grief
Is harsh and quite without relief:
Although I have not taken thirty silver coins,
I have through weary weakness,
Through my cowardly, confusing fault
Grown strangely blind.
I dare not go ahead
Nor can I now retrace
My steps,
Your Way I have no right to find
And I shall never see Your Face.

### DURING TREATMENT

Dear Doctor,

I desperately need to write so many things, but nothing comes when I sit down to do so. Even the verse I enclose which has been screaming to improve itself for days is not saying what I want it to say.

There is so much inside me that is despicable, and there is not even a strong desire to pray about it. I comprehend a great deal in my mind, and I might even carry it into my feelings, but I seem to be prevented—almost paralyzed. On the social surface I can manage quite nicely as is usually the case with me, but my true self is filled with confusion and the fear that it will never come right. I know that affirmation will come to me here or nowhere. I can trust you as I have never trusted anyone else. At the moment I find myself looking back at other persons I trusted at least in part, all of whom have in some way betrayed me. The confidence I feel in you is quite different and I know it is a *good*.

One line of the poem I read in your book really struck me today and I immediately identified with it:

"When bed time comes I kiss myself goodnight."

It still seems to me as if I should bear with myself and not bother others. I find myself over and over trying to hide what seems obnoxious within me by being loquacious and again "proving myself"—trying to "buy my way."

I feel as if I will come to a point where you will despise me as you get to know more about me, and yet I feel as if freedom will come to me only if I can explain and reveal things fully. I could not bear to have another door close.

Bitterly as I spoke in group last week, I know my community has given me far more than I ever deserved, and this adds to my sense of guilt so that it seems to roll up like a huge ball of tangled threads. Do you think I will ever extricate myself from all this? Why am I so childish? Today it seems as if the 47 years of *doing* has helped me to justify my existence, but just barely. I still feel as if I belong nowhere and that people accept me only with tolerance.

I know you speak only the truth to me, but do you really understand how bad I am? What part of me is saying all this? If I have a better self it is not evident to me today.

Am I taking too long to clarify my thinking and to find it possible to reach out for affirmation? At the moment I have no pity for myself. I hate so much in me and yet I do not want to be hated.

I do not know if any of this makes any sense.

### Group Therapy

Who am I?
Who am I?
How can I know
Looking from inside out,
Hearing from outside in?

I cannot stand apart
Unprejudiced, to recognize
To scrutinize,
Evaluate, interpret what I see.
How can I find the *me*
Objectively?
Each of you forms a surface
Which reflects
That I may see;
And yet each one deflects
The light in some strange way
To minimize, distort, or magnify,
Delineating now, today
How I appear.
There still remains a fear
That I must pose myself
As you determine I must be,
Strong for the strong
And weak unto the weak.
This is not what I seek.
I fight a half-blind pinioned self
Burdened with shields of sham,
With visions of the past futility
Of trying to speak true
Again I ask of you—
(Yet ultimate reply must come from me)
Who am I now?
When shall I really see?

*Journey—Continuing Destiny—Affirmation*

Must I be strong this time again
With that synthetic pseudo-strength
Composed of pride and loneliness and fear,
With that same longing to reach out,

Yet knowing someone else
Has greater need?

I have shown seeming strength
For just a little while.
May I be weak, however briefly now
So that the truth of my own long deprived
And fearful life
May draw from someone understanding
And a wealth of love?

Believe me, only thus
Can I begin to feel in me
A strength no longer ersatz or contrived,
Bedded within the soil
Of my weak self
Fostered and pruned
Held to the sun and rain.
O God! make me accept
However difficult
That which must come
Before I can be truly strong
To know
Acceptance and serenity
Assuring affirmation
Which is love.

### For My Doctor

It is only up the street that I must go,
Up the hill and across the way
And into the hearthplace of my home.
Why should it seem so far,
Why should a wind rise suddenly
Tearing with rough perfidity
Drawing me into heretofore unknown perplexity?

I had crossed nearly half a continent
In coming to this place,
Flown over oceans long ago in storm and fear,
Nearly met death in mountain hideaways,
Known what imprisonment and treachery could do,
Watched more than once a Phoenix rise for me and mine,
Packing up treasures now for one last walk
Across the deep red carpet I had chosen
For this haven of my ministry.

Here in my home with loved ones who so recently
Helped me break bonds of many years
To come this way:
Family of love and peace and indestructible fidelity
And happiness—
These I may hold and nurture and affirm
In truth, acceptance, loyalty and joy
Along the way of love.

Four others, though not family,
Have walked with me
Counting the few but heavy steps
Away from what the roadsign now so falsely reads,
Four who could see that walls which house duplicity
Must be vacated now.

They, too, have come with me
And I shall lead them
Unto the life they sought so vainly
In that other place.
They, too, have learned to watch
For gleaming sparks from ancient ashes of their lives;
They too will find
As from a death or seeming death
Their glowing Phoenix will arise.

### Affirmation

I had been halted in my search for Him
Who is my Goal, but Whom I feared as Goad.
Strange misconceptions made my hope grow dim;
Fear tortured me. I bore a crippling load
Of guilt that made me long to die
Because I could not shed nor longer bear
Nor further camouflage my pain, nor try
Again to find someone to care—to dare
To teach me how to readjust—to choose
What could be tossed aside, what might with joy
Be used to strengthen me; what I might lose,
What I might freely, utterly destroy.
Now I am loved, affirmed and understood
My searching self emerges true and good.

### AFTER TREATMENT

Dear Doctor:

When I left the affirming atmosphere of your home I felt optimistic and assured about my own growth in healing; yet I had certain misgivings about re-entry into the active religious life. Unfortunately the sisters in the convent where I had been assigned, although friendly, prayerful, and desirous of being helpful and understanding, were accustomed to an intensely active, work-oriented life; some of them in fact were of the "perfectionist" type. Because of my past conditioning in "buying my way," "carrying my load," "proving my worth" I found myself feeling very guilty when remarks were made about the amount of work being done by individual sisters, and the laziness of those who did not do their share. Certain sisters began to tell me how I could solve what they considered my "psychological problems." They had patterns for work and regulations for community living of which I was constantly reminded either by comment or by their setting an example.

After several weeks there I asked to go to a larger community where I hoped to find more freedom to be myself. Once again, I found that even in this group there was a constant "measuring" of how hard one person worked, how selfish another person was, and so on. Lists of so-called "volunteer committees" were posted on the bulletin board and those who did not feel able to sign for at least one of them were criticized at the next community meeting.

I was aware of a deep seated pattern with regard to this particular community where I had lived before and when I had always thought that I had to earn my right to live there by the work I did in both convent and school. In those earlier years I had had the health and strength to work hard and to please everyone in order to be accepted and make some real friends. Yet living there had never given me a feeling of home or "community," just a satisfaction from time to time that I was working hard enough to deserve my board, room and the necessities of life. All this had contributed eventually to my desperate need for healing, and I know I could not now, after having become a "psychiatric case," feel justified in considering myself a member of that house. My many chronic psychological ills were almost completely healed, but the attitude in these communities created still sufficient fear within me to prevent my putting into practice all I had learned from your therapy. The serious emergency surgery I required left me with neither the physical nor emotional strength to be the "real me" I had been led to discover while living in your home.

Thus the first four months after leaving you were bewildering and battling months. The new honest frankness I had learned and tried to practice was considered as selfish, critical, contradictory and "un-religious." My failure to explain, apologize, excuse, adapt was considered an un-pleasant reversal. My new decisiveness and my new efforts to go my own way were deemed to be stubbornness and secretiveness. I had been known as a person who was al-ways willing to change my plans for others, to explain and make excuses rather than have others think ill of me, to be smiling and pleasant at all times. I had been "condi-tioned" to jump to do things for others, to please them, never to criticize them or to assert myself in contradiction to their opinions, and I was chronically fearful of asking or accepting favors from anyone. In matters of obedience we had been taught to submit both our will and our judg-ment, and consequently I always had tried desperately to follow this plan through fear of displeasing God or man. Once again I began to despise myself and to take guilt upon my shoulders when deep down I knew it did not belong there.

I finally was able to move into an experimental thera-peutic house made up of sisters from my own religious community, and it looks as if they will support me in my determination not to allow my life to be ruled by guilt and fear as in the past. In this new community I see a genuine desire to respect each individual, to live like a family rather than an institute. Some of the sisters are working full time, some part time, some few are enjoying the freedom to find themselves in the atmosphere of this house and to consider new fields of work when they leave here. Haste, pressure, and incessant activity are not present. I am free now to do only as much as I feel able to do, and as my physical and emotional strength increase, I hope to find myself gradually woven into this community. Because of past pressures, and also because I have been interested in work that often requires concentration and quiet and opportunity for creative thought, I had often been inclined to find myself avoiding disturbing confron-tations, and excessive encroachments on my periods of work and study. In this group differences of temperament, age, interests, and patterns of living are understood and accepted.

Some religious orders, I realize, have been sadly remiss in providing psychiatric help for their sisters, and even those who have permitted it have failed to develop within the communities to which these sister-patients would return, any semblance of acceptance, understanding or affirmation. The patterns of religious life in the past have contributed to the development of the deprivation neurosis among religious sisters, brothers and priests. A deprivation neurotic in a therapeutic situation is living with others who have also been deprived of affirmation. These persons come to understand and appreciate one another. Being able to return to a truly affirming, as distinguished from a utilitarian, community is an integral part of the healing process. Just as a physical ailment requires convalescence under strengthening and appreciative conditions so does emotional illness. After a period of therapy for emotional illness there is all too often a quality of "re-entry" which is not present in a return for physical recuperation. Under such circumstances one of the first disturbing realizations will be that there is no one who talks the same language. The sense of one's own value as a person begins to fade from consciousness; the assurance of one's own abilities grows weak; an approach to social encounters becomes again more and more tentative and tenuous, and one becomes inhibited rather than outgoing. The resolution to speak openly about one's likes and dislikes; to express opinions assertively, yet calmly; to refuse to apologize or excuse when there is no call for apology or excuse; and the sincere effort to be one's real self without exaggerated efforts to please others, to win their favor, to avoid their anger, and so on—all these become increasingly difficult, if not impossible to adhere to. Yet, having learned to understand all these inherent problems, the deprivation neurotic knows that unless she can be free to carry out these resolutions with consistency and firmness she will fall back into the deeply depressive unhappiness of the past.

The group with whom I am now living have been together only a few months, but in that time they have learned much from each other both about one another and about themselves. They make sincere efforts to permit others to be "themselves"; they make allowances for one another, while at the same time when any sister wants help from the group they generously share their ideas and opinions. More communities of this type should help to spread a new understanding of the need for assertion rather than groveling compliance, the need to *be*, rather than to *do*, the need to be accepted as one is. Where disturbing human pressures are at a minimum, the mutually affirming members of the community learn the wisdom of leaving a very large part of the "personality remodeling" to the Holy Spirit. I am most grateful to my superiors for their pioneering work in setting up this non-utilitarian, affirming home and for the privilege of being allowed to complete here the healing process which began when I was put under your care a year ago.

### Departure from Babylon—Affirmation

Grasp now your harp
From where you hung it on the willow tree
For Babylon is falling:
Can you not see
That you are free?
Puny comforts of the land you leave—
Cast them from memory
Walk out in strength and now receive
All that awaits the daughters who believe.
So long you have not sung

A joyous song.
Driven by fear
Your harp was hung
Untuned, its listless strings
Incapable of sounding forth in joy.
You may destroy
False guilt of grief and wrong
That you endured.
Now you may be assured.
Wind tightly
On your harp each mute and loosened string;
Strike joyfully
That they may ring
And let your whole heart sing.

### Affirmation—The Coming of the Light

*Unto those who dwelt in the land of gloom*
*A light has shown*
Drawing them forth
To meet it on its way.
There is no further need
For them to heed
The heavy words that spoke their doom.
This is a bright new day.

*The yoke* that burdened them
Has been removed and cast aside.
*The rod* that marked
The tempo of each heavy task
Has stopped its beat.
There is no need to hide
Or to conform to those who ask
Them to repeat
Their years beneath a dark depriving cloud.
Now they may shout aloud,

As they move forward where the way is bright,
*"The people who walked in darkness*
*Have seen a great light."*

## *The Miracle of Affirmation*

So like a miracle—this rich new life
That came my way,
This warmth of clarifying light
That I enjoy today.
Seeking and searching I had run
So far astray,
All unbelieving
That these many years
I should have been quite free,
Receiving
Gift and grace to use, to show,
To build upon, to share.
I knew not where to go.
Because it seemed within me all had died
I wanted only some safe place to hide.
I thought no one could care
For me apart from goals I had achieved
Until one came who understood
And soon perceived
Beneath the actions credited to me
A strong desire for life
That could be genuine and free.
Accepting me unswervingly
With all the hidden growths
Within my soul
Of anger, loneliness, uncertainty,
Deep guilt and fear,
He found a way to clear
The agonizing jungle of them all
And drew me with a gentle call

Now to emerge wholeheartedly and free.
Trusting, patient, affirming, loving
He gave new life to me.

1—We came upon the following interesting item in the *New York Times*
Service of July 13, 1969, in regard to adults playing in a sandbox. We
leave it to the reader to draw his own conclusions.

New York, N. Y.—It was inevitable: the executive sandbox. And only
$465—(plus shipping from Toronto, Canada). Of course, the price in-
cludes duty and four bags of white Canadian sand.

The 15-inch-high, 42-inch-square plywood box, with teak, rosewood
or walnut veneer and fluorescent lighting concealed under a black plastic
sitting ledge, was the idea of Hugh Spencer, president and chief designer
of Opus International Ltd. He is billing his sandbox as "a creative piece
of furniture" and as "an excellent pacifier" for the tense businessman.

One pacified customer is Dr. Wilda Bynum, a counselor at the State
University of New York at Buffalo. She put the box in the middle of her
apartment living room and vouches for its therapeutic effects. "It's surprising how often I sit there and play in the sand," Dr. Bynum said.
"And when friends come, they all look for the best place to sit on the
ledge so they can play."

# CHAPTER IX

# WHAT DEPRIVATION NEUROTICS WRITE
## THEIR THERAPISTS

We want to share with our readers some insights gained from letters written to us by deprivation neurotic patients. More than anything else, these letters reveal glimpses of the suffering, fears, depressions, hopes, and longings of these patients.

> Dear Doctor, . . . for years I have been bothered a great deal with feelings of inadequacy. I feel so isolated, a nobody. I get depressed because I am so uninvolved and so small a person, so insignificant and unable to affect my environment. I have seen several psychiatrists but they do not seem to understand me. Recently I heard you lecturing about the deprivation neurosis and was overjoyed at learning that someone at last understands my illness. Just being enlightened on the matter has helped me a great deal already. I want to make an appointment with you as soon as possible.                    (from a male teacher)

> Dear Doctor, . . . It doesn't seem worth it to live another day. I want to die—there is nothing good to live for. I am ashamed to even walk out on the street. Ashamed and afraid. I am so afraid; at night it gets worse. Sometimes I rock in my rocker all night. Help me, this is torture. I don't want to be. I want to be like everybody else. Doctor, I got a little doll. It helps very much at night.

Also, because I get so afraid a small night light helps.

Thank you so much for letting me come to see you. It means a lot to me. You help very much. I've never been able to say much to anyone. But to you it is better; somehow you are easy to talk to.

I keep telling myself that somehow things will work out. But it is hard to trust that they will when God seems so unreal and religion something someone made up. But this makes me realize how really afraid of God I am. Just the idea of God caring for us, watching over us, our creator, our father, is repulsive. It is hard to say things. More so, I noticed, since I told you I want to die. It is frustrating not to express myself. It seems as though chains fall to the floor—just being with you.

> (from a woman religious, whose father
> had coerced eleven of his twelve children
> to enter the religious life)

Dear Doctor, . . . I am enjoying so many little things now and "not giving a darn" about the trivia that plague so many people! I feel I understand so much more of human life, and am getting closer to people, who, interestingly, seem to respond to this warmth. I really get a lump in the throat when I realize the tremendous depth with which one can sense and feel, and am shocked at how little it takes to become insensitive and unfeeling; I can really detect these periods and they are the unhappiest again, relatively.

The single most important idea I have learned from you is the one that suggests that one's basic instincts are positive and good, and that if allowed to rise to the surface will only result in good. I believe in this doctrine and until now it has been responsible for more happiness than any other single idea, for I now often simply "shoot from the hip," and darned if I'm not a better marksman than when I was always taking perfect aim!

What I also want to tell you is how important you have been in *allowing* me to make these changes. I purposely use the word allow because for me, at least, there was no frame of reference, no evaluator, to tell me what is permissible and what isn't. I am convinced that to ask a person to change his way of thinking and acting is the most optimistic gesture another man can make, because it is or was to me inconceivable that I could change. Hence, to me the patient's inability to conceive of himself as any person other than what he has been, is a singularly powerful force. You can call it resistance, or whatever formal name you wish, but the thought of being different from what I was, was not only impossible to visualize, but also risky, and for another person to say, "Go ahead . . . it's all right . . . nothing bad, only good, will happen," was just words. It was the constant encouragement and my perception that *you* really believed it that helped me to risk it, little by little.

(from a doctor of science)

Dear Doctor, . . . Yesterday I baby-sat for a little boy. He asked me, "Can't you come and stay here with me? You can play with me, you know." If he only knew how much I want to. It is so much fun in the sandbox, too. But don't tell anyone, Doctor.

(from a woman teacher)

Dear Doctor, . . . I still want my mother to hold me, but I won't admit it. In fact I feel it is immature and dirty, and besides she won't hold me anyway. I only come to see you, Doctor, because you hold my hand.

(from an airline stewardess)

Dear Doctor, . . . Maybe it is so difficult to express myself because I really don't know myself what I am like. I know I don't! So far my life has not meant anything to me . . .

I realize now that I must use my emotions, and not just knowledge alone. I know from what I've learned that the people who have the deepest and richest emotional potentialities are the ones that are most likely to suffer, while less sensitive people do not. It seems ironic that this is so . . . I have never counted what it costs to see you because it can't be measured by money. Nothing has ever meant as much in my life as knowing you. You are my model of a real man and complete person. I can sincerely even go this far: in every way but physically you are my father. For it is you who is teaching me what life truly means. You share my problems, something I never was able to do with my father. Physically and intellectually I am grown up, but emotionally I am yet like a child in your care. I will never be able to discharge my debt to you. I feel inside that you truly have the right answers. My childhood's experiences make it hard to trust anyone again, lest I might be on the wrong track again. I know you understand this. It has to be the right answer this time or else all will be lost. But slowly I have come to trust you and I know I am making progress, so you must be right.                    (from a male artist with super-
                    imposed, camouflaged fear-neurosis)

Dear Doctor, . . . I am afraid and want to die. I hate people. They can be so mean. They are always so busy, just doing things, going places, they think the only important thing is to be busy. To be busy about important things. How someone else feels or what he wants is not important to them. Children are more sensible than grown-ups. Grown-ups are too conceited and busy to have time for children.

Do you know what? The little children are coming from all around here and we're having a "doll-lawn-house and everything-party." They are so excited. The girls are bringing their dolls and the little boys are bringing their teddy bears and dogs and bunnies and storybooks I can read to them. It'll be a riot. I'll have so much fun.

People kind of push aside the children when they come, and call them pests. But they just want us to come down to their little world and show them you're a lot like them and they're so hungry for a little love and someone to laugh and play with them. God must love them. Children surely would go right to God if grown-ups would let them.                              (from a single woman)

Dear Doctor, . . . Tonight I've had it! We are a number, not a person. As I see religious life being lived, it's a big game of politics. As one sister who wanted to go to you, but was told to see another psychiatrist, said to me, the only time you get attention from your superior is when you want to leave the order or need psychiatric help. And then you are branded for life. Doctor, I've given and helped people all my life. Sometimes there is a deep hurt, a longing for someone to give in return and to accept and love you. If I told this to many of my fellow sisters I'd be told to grow up.                              (from a woman religious)

Dear Doctor, . . . I feel I am all alone and no one really loves or cares about me. Everything is a constant fight to hold on. My parents will not leave me alone, they do not listen to you when you explain the reason for my illness. They resent it. Lately my depression seems to get worse daily. All my life I have pushed myself, lived on will power, but I can't any longer. This is what I composed yesterday:

> You gave me something I have
>   not experienced with another:
> You said, "Sometimes it helps to
>   talk." Your hand closed warmly
>   on mine.

"Your hand is soft."
Gently you led me . . . Through a green
  countryside, warmed by soft
  summer breezes.

You spoke of tranquility . . . in
  gazing at a hill massed with
  trees.
You knew each bird—and the
  mustard seed.

It was as though you had known
  me before—each thought;
  the countless feelings swelling,
  and then the wonder and contentment.

I love the hollows in your cheeks, the
  clear greenish-blue of your eyes,
  the perception . . . the understanding,
  the calm sturdiness.

I will not consume you and destroy
  our yesterday. Patiently I will wait . . .
  but often put my head upon the table—
  in case you are there, and notice.
                    (from a single professional woman)

Dear Doctor, . . . My parents were absolutely determined
to control me regardless of my feelings. They were always saying, "You shouldn't *feel* that way . . . ," as though
I could change my feelings to suit their taste. It is so
horrible to be so misunderstood by one's parents all the
time. Doctor, I know I am terribly, terribly ill. I feel
sick unto death. I really do. I don't want to live. My
parents made it sound so wicked for me to have my
wants or desires, especially since I was prone to dance.

They told the principal of every school I went to that they did not believe in dancing and I had to sit on the side. Everything they stood for, with firm conviction, proved to me I did not belong. I knew I wanted different principles from them, theirs seemed so compartmented. Nothing was all of one piece for me, nothing fit. Religion said, "Be ye separate, 'Come out from among them. You are not of the world'." But to be in the world, and not of it, seemed so cruel, so painful, a deliberate attempt to make life impossible, which it was. We were to associate with only certain of the "born-again" ones—not even the Baptists, they were Calvinists! I am getting so I hate religion, it builds walls and separates people. I am weary of the strain of life; it is too much, really, all these demands to do good and right. I'd sure like to make some mistakes once in a while. It would beat the strain of being good and right all the time. That is just too much—even though I want to do right. I could not understand why all the kids found it so hard to stay on the straight and narrow. One simple word "No" was the answer. It was rather easy to say (especially if you are terrified of feelings, I guess).

Another thing—I loved to sing, but I was forbidden most of the worldly songs, and I had to confine myself mostly to religious songs, those that dealt with joy and love, and the rescuing of lost souls from sin and degradation. I tried so hard to believe the words, but they only depressed me. All this Christian "love and joy" was so depressing. My house is an unbelievable mess (the pictures her husband showed us one day proved the chaos in every room was simply indescribable!). My husband wants me to leave; he is depressed, discouraged, lifeless. Who wouldn't be after his wife has spent ten years in treatment with twelve or thirteen psychiatrists. I think I should go; I am no good to my lovely children, they deserve to love life, to find it rewarding and exciting. But I am afraid to be alone. I already feel afraid when I say the word "alone." I feel like I have been an orphan all my life, like I have been in a well-meaning foster home, but an unhappy one. I am an orphan. I don't belong anywhere. Ever since I was small my father said, "Never put your faith and trust in people; they will fail you and disappoint you. Keep your eyes only on Christ, only He will never fail. Friends will forsake you. Christ will never forsake you." The world was painted as such a wicked, terrible, threatening place all the time. Since this place is so wicked, why did God waste our time placing us here anyway? Everything has been so confusing, always. Confusion, confusion! . . . I remember how I would purposely do things to win adult smiles and attention, because I was so weary of disapproval! I knew perfectly how to get the whispered smiles, "Isn't that darling," etc.

Adults were so manipulatable; it was very disheartening and disappointing. It did seem to me adults were so awful. My feelings never did really matter. If I expressed a wish that "I don't like that" or some such statement, the reply was, "What? Why sure you do." Invariably, when engaged in some activity my parents didn't like, they would say, "You don't *want* to do that." Any time I voiced disillusionment I was promptly reminded of all my blessings as a little girl who had enough to eat, clothes on my back, and a roof over my head. We were repeatedly reminded of unfortunate children who did not have these things, and we were always made to feel guilty for wanting things. My father resented giving us things so much. His form of discipline was yelling all the time, denouncing our desires, and saying no to most things (unless *he* felt like doing it). It did not take long to learn that our desires were meaningless to him—it was what *he* wanted that counted. This hurts a child terribly . . . Doctor, this business of feelings being so important is beginning to make a new world for all of us here. It is such a tremendous change for me. I knew intellectually that feelings were important, but now it is sinking in, emotionally, gradually. When feelings are considered important, people are not so irritable and defensive. Each individual's feelings about himself, situations and others is important. It really is. Hooray! That is a most marvelous thing. Life for me has always been just following rigid rules, to do right; that was the only thing that counted. What a severe way to live. I have certainly hurt myself terribly by trying to give myself what I thought I deserved. But it has always seemed that everything natural for me to do or be, has been wrong in the eyes of my parents, and according to my own inferior self-image. No wonder nothing hangs together or makes sense. I am meant to be me. But who am I? Do I really have a right to be me?

My parents actually and purposely planned to break my will, so they could handle me. Mother told me when I was very little, "Parents have to break a child's will, or the child will be wayward and disobedient. It is not that we want to hurt you, but it must be done. We have seen the grief other parents suffer by spoiling their children with attention and we are not going to make that mistake." Then, of course, the Bible said explicitly, "Children, obey your parents in the Lord," so I did not have a chance, did I? I wanted to do right, but my feelings were so opposite to these teachings. Therefore it followed that I must be wrong. If my sincere Christian parents were not "in the Lord" nobody was! What a terrible freak I was, to want to do right with all my heart, yet to feel so opposite from my parents. Life and circumstances were filled with proof that I was the queer, stupid one. It was so wrong for me to have happy dreams —these were not meant for me. Adults were all domineering, I had to do things their way—there was no allowance for imagination. I could not understand how such a lowly hunk, a puny creature as I, was allowed to be born anyhow. It seemed to me that God was up there pulling strings, and just overlooked this dumb creature, but He would find me sooner or later and I would get my just deserts: doom! He could not possibly have any place for me. As a result I do not feel I belong anywhere. There is not a place in the world that is mine, and the sooner death overtakes me the better.

(from a mother of five children with superimposed, severe repressive neurosis)

Dear Doctor, . . . What a difference eighteen months of affirmation therapy have made in my life! I believe that after five years of psychoanalytic therapy and other forms of treatment by five psychiatrists and one psychologist I am well qualified to state that there is nothing like your therapy. I do not say that the other therapists didn't know their business, but they were trying to help me uncover repressed material while my basic problems had nothing to do with repression. They did not seem to realize that many of my deprivation neurotic symptoms resemble those of repressive neurotics and that you can be neurotic without repressions.

Since I moved to another state I have been more and more successful in daring to be myself. I continue to be surprised at how long it can take before one really feels what one has come to understand and accept intellectually, namely, that people have a right to be themselves. Or I should say that *I* have a right to be *myself*, because I have always believed that everyone else had that right except me. My parents and teachers in the seminary must have done a better than average job in making me a "thing," a robot, rather than a human being. They did everything to make me grow physically and intellectually, but they withheld the emotional food necessary to feel really worthwhile and lovable. No wonder I still feel like a boy; but that is progress for I was a baby when I first came to you.

Since I got rid of my "salt-and-pepper syndrome" (he never dared to ask people for such little favors as passing the salt for fear of displeasing them), I have been experimenting more in asserting myself in bigger things. Now that I consider my emotions my friends it is so much easier to bring up a contrary opinion in a conversation, to say 'no' when someone asks me to do something I don't care for. I feel much less tired now that I don't have to live only on one motor (will power), but am allowed to use also the motor of my emotions. Whenever I have a chance to take a walk in a forest, or, better still, along the ocean while the waves are smashing against the rocks, I scream at the top of my lungs. You remember how silly I felt when I first tried to do this at your suggestion, and how long it took me before I got over the fear of making a fool of myself, even when there was nobody around to see or hear me?

I no longer have a need to lend my support to some minority causes as I did five years ago, even to the point of being arrested and put in jail during a protest march. I still can't decide what was more important at the time: the feeling of being important because of getting TV coverage, which made up for my life-long feelings of inferiority, or the sense of belonging, of comraderie, that I felt when a group of us were plotting our strategy in protesting the Vietnam war or defying the IRS. I never had felt that I belonged anywhere, neither at home, nor in the seminary, nor in the rectories after I had been ordained. And when I took a leave of absence in order to join the peace movement I did it mainly to "get out from under"; I was sick of others having complete control over my life. Sure my parents, a nun-aunt, the rector of the seminary, my bishop and finally the pastors were always so nice in telling me what to do and how; it was always for *my* good, they said; but none had any idea of my need to be myself, to be a free, self-determining person who can be trusted to act in a responsible manner. I feel the Church and many of her representatives talk from both corners of their mouths. They say man has free will, but then proceed to scare him from early childhood with "you must do this, or else," and train him like an animal to perform certain acts regardless of his feelings.

Doctor, you have taught me what it really means to be a free human being—not that I'm quite free yet, but I know I'll get there some day—and to live by "I may," rather than by "I must." Hearing this over and over again in using your affirmation therapy tapes has greatly accelerated the process of liberating and integrating my emotions. And believe it or not, I still listen occasionally to our recorded therapy sessions. I am so glad you let me make these tapes. You always had so much to share with me that I could never have retained it all. Often I was so tense and nervous that I had forgotten half of what you had said by the time I left your office.

It feels so good to be more aware of my desires and to gratify them once in a while. And to feel happy at times without being plagued by feelings of guilt and thoughts of being selfish. I even experience extreme pleasure when I dare to think of *my* future as *I* want it— but it still gets squelched pretty fast by the ingrained memories of being told I must solely live to please others and God, never myself.

I know I still have some way to go, Doctor, but I no longer feel devastated when someone disapproves of something I do, or doesn't like me as much as I had hoped. Thus life is much more liveable than it was in the past, and it is wonderful to know that it will get even better. I am beginning to make friendships which are no longer solely on the terms of the other person. And I am sure that in the end Jesus will be my friend, too, even though my training for the priesthood, and the treatment received from well-meaning, but unaffirmed, overbearing superiors had succeeded pretty well in alienating me from the God I wanted to please and love from childhood. Church people have a lot to learn from you, Doctor; I hope and pray that they will study the books you and Dr. Terruwe have written, and will do everything in their power to repair the damage done in the past. What irony that they, "God's chosen ones," have contributed to so much unnecessary suffering among themselves and to the people they are supposed to lead to God. But I believe that things are going to be better in the Church. We hear more and more about a loving Christ who wants to heal everyone and have them live without fear. That is the very opposite of what I was taught, that it pleased God when we were sick and scared of Him.

I just wanted you to know that I am enjoying life more and that I am forever grateful for your opening the door of my prison.

(from a young priest, with a severe, super-imposed obsessive compulsive neurosis)

Dear Doctor, . . . I just saw your new book in a store and was so happy to see it contained your address. I lost track of your whereabouts since I moved to Arizona ten or eleven years ago. I have been so much happier since I got married to a very loving immigrant from Spain, also an artist, and was able to leave my non-affirming parents thousands of miles behind me . . . There is another thing that may interest you. You'll remember how I was made to speak Polish when a child by my smothering, fault-finding, scrupulous, punitive mother and my father who never dared to protect me from my mother's ravings and cruel and undeserved punishments. Well, I've forgotten the Polish language for all practical purposes, and even find it hard to speak English now that we live in a Spanish speaking community. Most people think that I was born in Spain or Mexico, and am trying to learn English! I don't care whether I forget my English, too, as long as my mother doesn't know how to speak Spanish. Even though I speak with her infrequently over the phone I have a feeling that she is now unable to invade my mind so to speak. It is as if my mind is one place she no longer can enter; it is like a wall that protects me from the endless prying she subjected me to since I was a baby. It gives me a privacy that I never had before. Unfortunately, thinking and speaking in Spanish doesn't afford protection against painful memories. In fact, when they are vivid as happens occasionally when I am depressed, I hear my mother shriek her accusations in a mixture of Polish, English and Spanish. It is awful. I am so glad I hardly ever see her.

(from a woman artist)

# CHAPTER X

# HOW TO PROTECT YOUR CHILDREN FROM BECOMING DEPRIVATION NEUROTICS

Just as the therapy of the deprivation neurosis differs decidedly from that of the repressive neuroses, so does its prevention. Elsewhere we have explained that the prevention of repressive neuroses center around several interrelated factors in man's sensory, intellectual, and spiritual lives. In deprivation neurosis, prevention deals with a single factor; namely, mature, unselfish love and its affirming, creative effect on a human being. The actual prevention of deprivation neurosis is not necessarily simpler than that of the repressive neuroses. For though it is relatively easy to understand the fundamental principle, its application in everyday life is far more difficult. Witness the great and ever-growing number of unaffirmed people in our society who suffer from a full-blown deprivation neurosis, or lead unhappy, lonely, insecure lives, not knowing why they suffer from recurring depressions, irritability, chronic alcoholism, chronic fatigue, or vague physical complaints which respond to medical treatment only temporarily, if at all.

The ease with which we grasp the principles involved in the prevention of these neuroses is in inverse ratio to their ease of application. The prevention of repressive neuroses depends largely on our doing things which we have learned are proper and correct. These things chiefly require intelligence and good will. But in the prevention of deprivation neurosis and its sub-clinical states of non-affirmation, the emphasis lies on a state of *being* for and with another, of being moved inwardly by his goodness and unique worth prior to *doing* anything for him. We have already referred to this in the chapter on the therapy of deprivation neurosis, warning against therapeutic manifestations of love for the patient that are not sincerely felt.

NATURE OF HUMAN LOVE

We cannot present here a complete and detailed study of the psychology and philosophy of human love. But we will select those aspects of it which deal with the relationship between the adult and the developing human being, the already affirmed person and the not yet affirmed one, the mature and the immature, the parent and the child. These aspects are: 1) the requirements of this love on the part of the parent; and 2) the action of this love on the child.

From the very first day of extrauterine life the infant needs to experience genuine unselfish love from another human being if it is to attain the fullness of its human existence and authentic happiness; that is, the joy which is the fruit of loving and being loved. This love, of course, has nothing to do with sexuality, the all-pervasive influence of Freud's theories notwithstanding. The only reference to sex which would be warranted in this context is that of gender sex, of masculinity and femininity, in that man or woman, father or mother, express love for their children in different ways. Truly mature human love is a combination of *emotional and volitional love*. The feeling or emotion of love is a movement or arousal of our sensory nature by the good which attracts us. Volitional love is the movement of the will towards that same good or, in this discussion of love between people, towards the well-being and happiness of the other. Even in the absence of feelings of love, the will, moved only by the intellect, can still bring about all the external acts of love. It is this love of the will, and only this love, which is the object of every commandment dealing with love, whether for God, one's parents, one's neighbors, or one's enemies. If it so happens that the feeling of love participates in, and in turn, moves volitional love, it will be accompanied by great joy and satisfaction, but such feeling cannot be commanded.

When both emotional and volitional love readily interact, and acts of love proceed from the two together, we experience genuine, mature human love. Our volitional love provides us with the spiritual gladness of being directed toward what is truly good in itself, for instance, God. But only when the feeling of love fully partakes of this process do we also experience "sensory gladness," the feeling of joy. Together, spiritual and sensory gladness constitute the happiness for which man is created, "for which man strives naturally and by necessity," as Aquinas said.

It is precisely this genuine, mature human love, this mixture of constantly interacting emotional and volitional love, which the child requires throughout its development in order to become who he is, to relate confidently to others, to cope adequately with the stresses of life, and to enjoy its goodness and beauty. Moreover, by receiving this love the child grows up ready to love others in turn and—in the fullest sense far transcending the merely physical procreative act—to create children.

In this discussion of integral human love we particularly stress the emotional aspect for two reasons. First, because more than the volitional aspect, it belongs to the psychotherapist's field of competence. Second, because in a way it needs our more thoughtful attention, especially when compared with the volitional aspect which determines the moral value of an act and therefore has been taught and stressed extensively throughout the ages by the Church and moral theologians. While we shall never divorce the two aspects of human love in our discussion, we shall consider the love of the will only insofar as it influences the operations and expressions of emotional love.

#### LOVE—A PSYCHOPHYSICAL REACTION

Understood in this way human love is evidently a psychophysical event with its own psychomotor reaction, i.e., the somatic reaction of a psychic event. The somatic changes are as much an integral part of the emotion of love as the generally better-known somatic reactions of rapid heartbeat, dry mouth, and cold and trembling hands and feet are part of the emotion of fear. These somatic reactions, though in essence the same for all individuals, differ somewhat in the manner of expression depending on such factors as gender, race, temperament, and psychic disposition. For example, a woman's psychomotor reaction of love usually occurs sooner and with greater intensity than that of a man. Mediterranean people differ similarly from the Scandinavians.

### TENDERNESS

The most typical characteristic of mature human love is tenderness, whether manifested in the tone of voice, words, touch, or the way one looks at the beloved. One is tender because one senses the other's goodness and beauty, because one realizes how precious he is. One takes care to let the other be as he is, precisely because one loves him just the way he is at that moment. One is happy to be with the other, taking nothing for oneself, attempting no changes or accomplishments. One is respectful of the other's intrinsic goodness; never demanding, aggressive, or possessive.

It is through the tender *touch*, the tender look, the tender words and tone of voice that the child is affirmed in its own goodness, worth, and lovableness. The tenderness with which a mother cradles her infant in her arms, cuddles and caresses it, and presses it to her, is as primary in the order of importance as it is in the order of development. Without such tactile expressions of maternal love the child will develop later in life the most serious form of deprivation neurosis.

The infant is so highly sensitized through the most sensitive of its sense organs, the sense of touch, that we know of deprivation neurotic women who, they have been told, pushed their mothers away at a very early age, presumably because they could sense the willed or possessive character of their mothers' caresses. Interestingly, in all these cases the mothers, being deprivation neurotics themselves, stopped cuddling and caressing their babies, interpreting this behavior as a rejection of themselves. Tenderness, obviously, cannot be willed. It is the emotional expression of the feeling that the other is good, lovable, and a source of delight precisely as he is.

Similarly, such tender love leaves its unmistakable mark in the expression of the *eyes*. The tender gaze is characterized by repose and tranquility in the delight of contemplating the good. It reflects admiration and awe, as well as the joy of love. It changes in character as soon as one feels a desire to possess or direct the other to oneself. Nor does the other fail to sense this, for the will can mask or control the expression of the eyes only very slightly, certainly less than it can influence the tactile sense, and far less than it can words. This may be due partly to the fact that people are very little aware of the way in which their eyes mirror their inner feelings.

The third way that a child can and needs to experience its own goodness and thus the feeling of self-worth is through gentle *words* of love and a tender *tone* of voice. Whereas the tone of voice is wholly determined by one's feelings of love and only with effort susceptible to the influence of the will, words of love are readily spoken by an act of the will alone. Yet a sensitive person, especially one much in need of genuine love, such as a baby or other nonaffirmed person, can readily sense that such words are not authentic, that they do not proceed from a feeling of delight in him as a lovable object.

## AFFIRMATION

Genuine human love, manifesting itself in tenderness toward the child, is of primary importance for the developing psychic life. Only genuine love declares unequivocally to the child that the other has recognized him as good and valuable. Only this love affirms the child's goodness and worth, and because this process takes place on the emotional level, in the sensory sphere, it becomes anchored in the soma, in the biological organism where it forms a lasting source of the feeling that the child is a good for himself as well as for others. Without it he may in later years arrive at the conclusion that he is good because of what he does: performing his duties, showing obedience, getting good grades at school, attaining success in his profession, and so forth. Yet this cognitive knowledge will never provide him with the feeling of self-love which is the indispensable requirement for the fullness of his existence as a social being. "Man's being," says Heidegger, "is to be with others," to commune with one's fellow men in a union of feelings, of mutual emotional rapport. Man's nature as a social being absolutely demands this emotional *contact* with others. However, he can not become open to others unless he has first been affirmed by another's unselfish love. Without such affirmation he is doomed to a life of gnawing uncertainty about his own self-worth. No degree of professional or intellectual accomplishments, however outstanding and widely acclaimed, can make up for this emotional deficit. It can only be filled by the unselfish love of another person.

It is remarkable that the affirming character of mature human love has received relatively little recognition except for the *maternal deprivation syndrome*, in which its importance has been limited to its effect on the baby. When we discovered the syndrome of deprivation neurosis, we became convinced that affirmation is of universal significance for all human beings regardless of their age. It is the soul of love's fruitfulness. First, because it enables the other to become what he is destined to be, himself and no other. Second, because it affirms the other whether he reciprocates or not. The gift of affirmation together with its creative effects are his forever regardless of his response to the giver. Third, because ordinarily it awakens in the one affirmed a reciprocal love for the giver. Through this love he affirms the giver in return. In mutual love and oneness of feeling they experience the greatest human joy and the ultimate fulfillment of their natures.

Nevertheless, it is possible that affirmation will not lead to reciprocal love when, for instance, the other is innately incapable
of loving or possesses a certain antipathy toward the giver which
is not compensated for or relieved by his love. It is also possible
because an irrational fear or an excessive utilitarian drive stands
in the way. Whatever the cause, the giver suffers the pain of
unrequited love. For a deeply sensitive person this can be the
profoundest of all suffering.

### SELF-RESTRAINING LOVE

We stated above that the process of affirmation, so necessary
in the prevention of deprivation neurosis, is primarily one of
*being,* and secondarily of *doing,* of being loving and, secondarily,
if at all, performing certain acts of love. But acts of love may
under certain circumstances be harmful. Indeed, we claim that
doing little or nothing at all when the well-being of the other
requires this may be the very proof of the maturity of one's love.
Unfortunately, self-restraint in this context is often mistaken
for neurotic repression and consequently is not practiced. To
clarify the *difference between repression and restraint* in the
matter of love we should recall that every emotion tends toward
its sense object and simultaneously toward respectful and considerate guidance by reason. Therefore, when an emotion arises
which reason, not fear, decides should not be allowed to be gratified for the sake of another greater good, restraint must be exercised in the expression of this emotion without interfering with
the experiencing of the emotion itself. If this is not done, the
ensuing act, although providing a certain emotional gratification,
will not be a rationally human act and therefore will generate
disharmony in the psychic life. The other possibility is that fear
or energy prevents the emotion from running its course by repressing it. Neither process is correct: in the former, reason is
frustrated, in the latter, the emotion.
    All this we discussed at length in the original edition in our
treatment of repressive neuroses, although we never applied it

specifically to the emotion of love. What we said then about feelings of hate, anger, and sex holds equally for the first and foremost emotion of man's psychic life. *One must never repress the emotion of love.* Like all the emotions, love is an intrinsic and necessary good which must never be dealt with in an unnatural manner. It must always be felt and experienced, whether it is to be expressed or not. One is often aroused by love toward a sense object which, if allowed to run its full course, would not constitute a rational good. If this object were another human being, any number of circumstances could make it improper and imprudent to display one's feelings of love in a certain manner. Reason and will then require that one refrain from letting the feeling of love proceed beyond this stage. Although this means that one will not attain the joy of possessing the loved object, one will experience in its stead a much more profound yet at the same time *more spiritual feeling of joy,* because one's love has been shown in a truly noble and unselfish way through self-restraint, not repression. This more spiritual joy will perhaps not come readily to persons of a predominantly sensory orientation toward life. However, this would merely indicate the presence of a psychic deficiency in such people, for it is characteristic of the truly mature man to find his greatest joy and happiness precisely in the nobler, more spiritual things of life. The more a person has attained to spiritual maturity, the more he will comprehend the joy of this self-restraining love and his love will then be more truly love of another. In fact, one might well *measure the degree of unselfishness* of one's love of another by the degree and depth of the inner joy and happiness one derives from this self-restraining love.

When a person refrains from displaying his love because it would not be good for the other, he sacrifices the desire of his own love to the well-being of the other. This indeed is the *highest form of love.* It would be even nobler if, for the sake of the other and his rational good, the display of love were restrained, however difficult this is to do, even though such a display might be good for the other's emotional life and desired

by him. Anyone of adequate experience knows that the glory
of love does not lie in its abundance, but rather in the measure
and manner of bestowal adequate for the other and in the joyful
experiencing of the self-restraint which human love demands.

### INDICATIONS FOR SELF-RESTRAINING LOVE

The need for self-restraining love may be twofold. First,
when objectively considered, a particular manifestation of love
is not a reasonable good—if, for instance, it calls for actions which
conflict with the objective moral order. Second, when, subjectively considered, the one loved is psychically incapable of a
proper response to a certain manifestation of love.

The former is especially true in the *sexual manifestations* of
one's love. Since the objective moral order is identical with the
subjective good of oneself and others, the love which leads to
acts which are in conflict with this order cannot be mature. The
feeling of love which inclines a person to sexual acts is not, of
course, wrong in itself. It is a perfectly natural psychic response.
Yet volitional love calls for restraint of the emotional love lest
it issue in objectively wrong actions. The currently all-too-
popular thesis that all is fair in sexual behavior when it is prompted by feelings of love, is in conflict with the most elementary
rules of human relationships. Only volitional love illumined by
reason can provide the proper norm. Only living in accord with
this norm, which demands self-restraint, fulfills human nature
and provides the most profound happiness.

A very beautiful example of this was given by a young
farmer who had hoped to get some medication from us because
he could not control himself properly in the presence of his
fiancee. "My girl is so sweet and beautiful. I am crazy about her,
but I just can't keep my hands off her." His outlook on life was
healthy and mature and we were impressed by his noble character and sensitive appreciation of human love. He had no difficulty in understanding that his desire to fondle the girl was perfectly natural, and that he could demonstrate his unselfish love

for her in the most beautiful and authentic way by restraining himself in the expression of his desire. He left us happy with this newly discovered insight, and returned three months later enthused about the beauty of its application. "You know, Doctor, you really taught me something wonderful. It has made us both so happy! Why didn't anybody tell us that before? We are almost sorry that we won't have to do this anymore once we are married!"

The other need for self-restraining love derives, as we said, from considering the subjective needs of the other. In mature love one first seeks the good of the other and takes care that the manifestations of one's love are suited to the level of the other's psychic development. This applies first of all to all individuals whose emotional lives are not yet integrated with their rational faculties, either because they are infants, children, or adolescents, or because they are adults in whom the development of this integration was delayed or arrested. Certain manifestations of love which are good in themselves are not good for these individuals if they cannot respond to them in a reasonable manner. Almost every mother exercises this self-restraining love quite naturally and spontaneously toward her child. On the other hand, too many parents give their children too many and too expensive toys too early, before the children have had the opportunity to develop a strong desire for them. The failure of these parents to properly restrain their love results in the children becoming spoiled.

Adults too need to practice self-restraint in their love for one another. No matter how much two persons love each other, their emotional lives are not perfectly attuned at all times. Hence the need to be considerate in the moment and the manner of expressing one's love so that it will be good for the other to experience it. *Self-restraining love is the natural perfection of human love* because it is concerned exclusively with the good of the other, to the exclusion, if need be, of one's own.

Some will raise the question: Is this perfection psychologically feasible, and will this self-restraint in practice lead to a repression of the feeling of love? The answer is simple if one recalls that *every emotion in striving for its object also has an innate need to be guided by reason.* Such guidance, therefore, can never lead to psychologically abnormal consequences. If repression of the feeling of love occurs anyway, it never belongs to the nature of self-restraint. It is a mistaken attempt at attaining self-restraint, and the cause lies elsewhere.

On the other hand, it is to be expected, especially in the earlier phases of maturing, that one will make mistakes in the exercise of self-restraint simply as a result of the imperfection of human nature. Like everything else in nature, growth toward integrated emotional and volitional love takes time. One should not become disturbed by these failures in restraining oneself, but dare to accept them as virtually inevitable consequences of our fallible human condition. As long as one's will is well directed, one can proceed with the confidence that in time one will succeed.

### SELF-AFFIRMATION

By far the greatest obstacle in this maturing process lies in the unaffirmed person himself. His condition prevents him from affirming others, even his spouse and children. In this sense it must be considered a self-perpetuating emotional illness in spite of all attempts at arresting it by *self-affirmation.* This, we believe, is one of the major contributing factors in the increasing unrest in the world, especially in our sensate occidental culture in which man rushes headlong from one pleasure to the next without ever finding tranquility and peace. Some unaffirmed people seek to affirm themselves in sexual promiscuity and the pursuit of various sensate pleasures. Others try to impress the world with their importance by amassing material riches, by excessive striving for achievement in work and community affairs, or through the acquisition of status symbols ranging from cars to academic degrees. Some seek power over others in politics, or become aggressive, even homicidal, toward their fellow men.

But all attempts at self-affirmation are futile.[1] Even attempts to escape from the psychic prison of non-affirmation by mind-expanding drugs are doomed to fail. Only other human beings, not things or symbols, can unlock this prison, can disclose one's human goodness to oneself and others. The unaffirmed person, who doubts his self-worth and does not know who or what he is, tries to hide this from others by wearing a mask and playing a role. Many become expert at pretending to be what they are not. The more energy they spend in this way, the more fatigued they become, the more they isolate themselves from others and also from themselves.

Only when the unaffirmed person is unselfishly loved by another will he dare to lower his mask little by little, to play his role less rigidly in the realization that he is allowed to be what he really is; in this way he will find new strength and energy, will breathe more easily in the enlarging psychic sphere he shares with the other, and thus will find joy in living. Without the loving other, life has little significance for the unaffirmed person locked within himself, and he can mean but little to others. The suffering of the unaffirmed person was well described by Jean-Paul Sartre, himself without a father and raised as an only child by a childlike mother, when he wrote, *My loneliness is my prison, my punishment for a crime I am not aware of.*

## NON-AFFIRMATION AND NON-ASSERTIVENESS

Unaffirmed persons learn early in life to refrain from asserting themselves for fear of not being loved. Thus they make it their business to consciously suppress and not express their angry feelings. Such *suppression* may become readily enforced by *repression* of these same emotions, especially when these persons meet with other reasons for fearing anger, annoyance, hate and so on. This may happen as the result of certain religious teachings; of training based on human respect rather than objective moral standards; the unreasonable punishment of angry behavior or the reversal of parental roles. Except for those who set out to affirm themselves in various assertive and even aggressive ways, unaffirmed individuals become emotionally cripples and socially ineffective and pathetically self-effacing through the suppression of the emotions which serve their innate assertive drive: courage and anger. Thus an unaffirmed person frustrates his drive and need to be his unique self, his drive towards self-realization and self-preservation through assertiveness and competitiveness, and by overcoming obstacles and threats against one's life and welfare. Such a handicapped person is often advised to become more aggressive. Yet this is psychologically and therapeutically unsound advice. For *man is by nature not aggressive*, i.e., according to Webster, "tending to, or characterized by a first or unprovoked attack, or act of hostility; the first act of injury leading to a war or controversy."

"Assertive" is defined by Webster as, "characterized by, or disposed to affirm, to declare with assurance, to state positively; to maintain or defend, e.g., one's rights or prerogatives." Thus it would appear that an innate drive to defend oneself (assertion) is more properly expressive of man's nature than a drive to attack without provocation (aggression). Similarly, the emotion of anger serves the purpose of arousal toward overcoming obstacles and defensive action against danger (assertion), and not toward a first, unprovoked act of hostility or injury (aggression) in the absence of a danger. It definitely makes for a sounder psychology to make this clear distinction between assertion and aggression. And in therapy, too, it makes more sense to help the patient to become more assertive rather than more aggressive. Neurotic patients are more willing to cooperate in the former endeavor, but resist the latter.

The chronic suppression and non-use of the emotions which serve man's assertive drive has the most serious repercussions on the individual himself as well as on society. The individual is unable to be himself and to freely and spontaneously pursue his goals by means of an easily controlled, readily guided assertiveness. He is unable to love and be loved which, contrary to popular belief, is not so much the consequence of hate but rather of his enforced self-centeredness and imprisonment within himself. He cannot find joy in living and is subject to deep depressions and psychosomatic disorders. He is subject to uncontrollable outbursts of anger or rage against those who failed to affirm him and thus caused him to experience himself as unlovable, without worth, evil. We are inclined to believe that there exists a direct relationship between the rising suicide rate among young people and the rate of crimes of violence on the one hand, and the fast growing number of unaffirmed persons and deprivation neurotics in our society on the other.

## ALCOHOLISM AND NON-AFFIRMATION

Insofar as we can judge, the increase in the number of unaffirmed people is frightening. One would be hard put to count them all, but it would be no surprise if they represented a fourth of the population of the Western world. Among them we would have to include a large percentage of chronic alcoholics. There have been many unaffirmed people and deprivation neurotics among our alcoholic patients, and we have been struck repeatedly by the reports of authors, who, in attempting to describe an "alcoholic personality," almost always mention the main symptoms of the syndrome of deprivation neurosis. To quote, for example, from a recent psychiatric study which describes a characteristic life style, rather than specific personality traits of the alcoholic: "A deeply felt sense of inadequacy is invariably present . . . the earliest memories center on damage or abandonment, and the reaction of helplessness . . . a distinctive *hypersensitivity* is present, especially noticeable in personal relationships and in attitudes about talent, creativity, and success. Achievement is frequently discounted and is not experienced as success or as the fulfillment of genuine ambition . . . compensates for his deepening sense of inadequacy by ascribing to himself special qualities or talents, and by setting grandiose goals to prove that he is worth more than others think. . . ."

And from a widely circulated book by a recovered alcoholic

and respected member of Alcoholics Anonymous we quote: "He has been too dependent throughout his life on some person . . . feels insecure, incompetent and childlike . . . essentially a lonely class of people . . . anxious, fearful and tense in the real world . . . can't stand reality . . . is guilt-laden and rigid . . . takes the joy out of everything he does . . . the central desire of his whole nature is that of being caressed by his mother . . . the source of his craving for attention is often a lack of self-confidence . . . failure to accept and love himself. . . ."

The relatively few remaining personality features in this particular chapter, not quoted here, are typical of alcoholic repressive neurotics, and another few of alcoholics with psychopathic personality disorders. This corresponds to our clinical impression that the largest percentage of alcoholics is made up of unaffirmed people with or without a superimposed repressive neurosis; the next smaller group consists of individuals with a repressive neurosis; and by far the smallest group is comprised of psychopathic personalities who, of course, have little or no need to seek relief from alcohol since they suffer very little tension or anxiety. Somewhere between the last two groups are so-called normal people without significant emotional conflicts who become alcoholics after years of steady social drinking. Their personality characteristics, being average and thus *normal*, will not show up in an attempted description of an alleged alcoholic personality.

Being familiar with the various types of neuroses enables one to make sense out of a rather bewildering array of personality characteristics attributed to the alcoholic. Moreover, insights based upon this classification complement the A.A. approach to the disease of alcoholism, pointing out the need not to treat all alcoholics according to the same principles, except, of course, those pertaining to alcoholics as sick human beings with a common addiction. Beyond the A.A. approach which represents a combination of *will training* and a certain degree of *mutual affirmation*, alcoholics require specific psychiatric treatment if they are to enjoy lasting sobriety. Interestingly, the distrust, if not complete rejection, by many A.A. members of psychoanalytic therapy for alcoholics finds its justification in our understanding of the different types of neuroses. If our opinion is correct that psychoanalysis is indicated only in hysterical neurotics, who constitute a very small percentage of repressive neurotics, and, of course, an even smaller percentage of all neurotics, it follows that only a very small number of alcoholics could be expected to benefit from this type of psychiatric treatment.

The unaffirmed and deprivation neurotic alcoholic needs, in addition to active membership in A.A., one kind of psychotherapy; the repressive neurotic another; some alcoholics require a combination of both; and the *normal*, not-emotionally-disturbed alcoholic requires only the straight A.A. involvement directed at total abstinence. The psychopathic alcoholic, of course, will rarely benefit from any form of treatment for a prolonged period of time.

Recognition of these therapeutic needs would no doubt boost the present recovery rate of the A.A. program and provide a basis for a more circumspect application of its will-training aspects, especially regarding the alcoholic obsessive-compulsive neurotic. There seems to be every indication that the welfare of alcoholics would be served by a *rapprochement* between Alcoholics Anonymous and non-psychoanalytical psychiatry. Each discipline stands to benefit from the other in various ways. For example, anthropocentric psychiatry from A.A.'s philosophy of man's dependence on a power greater than himself, and A.A. from a more profound psychological understanding of normal and emotionally ill man.

The success of the A.A. program insofar as it finds its source in its affirming element is further proof of all people, not only professional people, possessing definite potentialities for affirmation.

To be sure, the psychiatrist will be engaged for a long time to come with the therapy of the many deprivation neurotics whose condition has gone unrecognized for so long. But ordinary people can do much to alleviate the suffering of their unaffirmed neighbors. Since they have to know what affirmation is and how to practice it, they must be taught by word and example. We think here particularly of the important role which awaits the representatives and followers of Christ, the perfect affirmer of men.

Judging by the accounts of the news media during the last several years, one is generally inclined to put much of the blame for the multi-faceted suffering of unaffirmed people on society, politicians, poverty, unfair discrimination, housing shortages, and so on. One expects government welfare programs, increased expenditures, improved living quarters, and so forth to be a panacea for this suffering. To the extent that these ills and remedies are not related to non-affirmation, they do not concern us here. But to the extent that they do, we may ask if rich people suffer less from nonaffirmation than the poor. If they did, we would not observe this syndrome of deprivation neurosis in the well-to-do. Yet the opposite is true. Nor is it difficult to diagnose this syndrome with a great likelihood of accuracy in public figures, especially those in the entertainment world. Not a few of them have proved this diagnosis correct through their untimely deaths at their own hands. Some may object that it is necessary to provide better housing for tense, depressed mothers of small children living in oppressive quarters before affirmation can exert its possible beneficial effects. The answer to this objection is that such women are not capable of finding joy and tranquility in more favorable surroundings and prosperity as long as they are not affirmed, and they will, therefore, remain isolated and lonely within themselves. On the other hand, once affirmed, they could cope much better with limited resources, sharing their own inner joys with those of others in spite of the shortcomings of their milieu.

ABORTION ON DEMAND AND AFFIRMATION

In relation to mothers and their children we are reminded of another group of human beings direly in need of affirmation;

namely, the unborn. The destruction of innocent human life is the most extreme form of non-affirmation. Its effect on the mother is no less grave, since she destroys the very being which is destined to affirm her in its own unique way. As the Dutch physician-poet Van Eden wrote, "He sent it back to us, our sign of love." The smile of the infant is the first and certainly not the last affirmation of its parents. Abortion is a form of psychic self-destruction, and if practiced on a large scale it will have the gravest consequences for any society which condones it. Abortion is an act of aggression, not an assertive act. (see p. 191).

Those who advocate abortion on demand often assert that there are already too many unwanted children in the world. This claim is in complete agreement with what we have discussed in this chapter; there are too many mothers who, not having been affirmed themselves, are incapable of affirming their children. We have already stated that abortion is the ultimate denial or non-affirmation of both fetus and mother, so it cannot be the answer to this very real problem. What help is there then for an unaffirmed pregnant woman? Nobody will dispute that to be effective, any help must aim at the well-being of the one in need of help; that is, such help must issue from unselfish love. But the essence of this love is affirmation. Therefore the question must be formulated, "How is a pregnant woman to be affirmed?" For the sake of clarity we shall distinguish between the pregnant woman who has been affirmed, and the one who has not.

For the woman who has been affirmed and therefore is capable of disclosing to her child its own worth, help that is worthy of the name of affirmation means assisting her to be who she already is. It means helping her to be the one who can and wants to affirm her unborn child by loving it tenderly. Affirming her child consists in the mother's protecting it in the unborn state and in due time leading it safely into the world. Helping this mother can never be advising or demanding that she have an abortion.

In the case of a pregnant woman who was never affirmed herself, we are dealing with a person who through no fault of her own is incapable of affirming her child. For her too, unselfish help consists in her being affirmed. This is done by assuring her that she is not guilty of being unable to affirm her child, and that nobody expects this from her. Real affirmation means letting her know that she can rely on the help of others in her situation of dependency and impotence. With this unselfish help she can rise to the point of affirming her unborn child herself by protecting it from harm, and later by delivering it from its dark enclosure. Not to help her in this way, but to advise her to abort, is to *deny* her—the very opposite of affirmation—and to push her even deeper into her loneliness and isolation, to provoke a depression which in our experience is malignant and incurable.

### WAYS OF AFFIRMATION

We close this chapter with a word of encouragement to all who are desirous of affirming their fellow men but do not know how to do so. For many, the first step often has to be a negative one; namely, not doing the opposite, something most of us seem to do so readily, however well-intentioned. Examples are criticizing, nagging, fault-finding, belittling, pointing out and reminding one of past mistakes and present shortcomings. These acts are direct and explicit denials of the other's goodness. Telling the sad and crying boy to be brave, to wipe his tears and think of all the children who are so much worse off than he; giving words of advice too quickly without being sensitive to the feelings behind a question—such are examples of subtle denial under the guise of kindness and encouragement. But all these are only the extremes in a wide range of possible forms of denial.

For others again the initial step has to be a desisting from their attempts at self-affirmation. No matter what the nature of their self-affirmation may be, it leaves no room for affirmation of their fellow men.

The next step is to learn to become more open and sensitive to what is already good in the other, and to express one's approval and admiration for this goodness in ways that will arouse feelings of pleasure in the other's recognition of his own goodness and worth. At the same time one must be willing to wait for, and to help, if need be, in the growth of still imperfect things toward their fulfillment and completion. Through one's constant affirmation and patient presence, the other grows in strength and courage to make these other things become good.

The ways of showing one's approval and encouragement are infinite. They range from cheering on one's favorite football team and applauding the concert pianist at the end of his performance to the beautiful and subtle examples of affirmation in the life of Christ. The New Testament is replete with them. Instead of denying the Samaritan woman at the well by not associating with her as a Jew would, Christ affirmed her when he said to her, "Give me a drink of water" (Jn 4:9). He affirmed the senior tax collector whom everyone considered a sinner with the words, "Zacchaeus, come down, hurry, because I must stay at your house today" (Lk 19:5).

On the occasion of his baptism Christ was affirmed when a voice came from heaven, "Thou are my beloved son; in thee I am well pleased" (Lk 3:22). And was not even the risen Christ asking for affirmation when he asked Simon Peter three times, "Simon, son of John, do you love me more than these others do?" and Peter answered him three times, "Yes, Lord, you know I love you" (Jn 21:15-17). And is it not true that at the Last Judgment, when our Lord sees and presents to us what is good in us, that He will free us from our prison of self-condemnation with the words, "For I was sick and you visited me, in prison and you came to see me" (Mt 25:36).[2]

1—Wholesome self-affirmation is possible only for the person whose emotional and intellectual integration is already well on its way to completion. We want to alert the reader to Rollo May's use of the term self-affirmation in his book *Power and Innocence.* His is distinctly different from ours and therefore creates confusion. This has been discussed in more detail in *Born Only Once* by C.W. Baars, M.D.

2—For an easy-to-read discussion of affirmation, non-affirmation, self-affirmation and pseudo-affirmation the reader is referred to the illustrated book, *Born Only Once,* by Conrad W. Baars, M.D., Franciscan Herald Press, Chicago, Ill., 1975.

# EPILOGUE

AFFIRMATION OR SELF-AFFIRMATION?

*A Crucial Question!*

It was in 1960 that our first brief clinical description of a newly crystallized neurosis, not caused by repression of the emotions, appeared in the English psychiatric literature.[1] In the years that followed we have become increasingly concerned with the diverse and far-reaching consequences of the lack of affirmation, the root cause of what we have called the deprivation- or frustration-neurosis, on individuals and society in general. Indeed, this latter effect on society must, in our opinion, be considered alarming, the more so since few people seem to be aware yet of the cause and effect relationship between the behavioral patterns of unaffirmed individuals and such manifestations as polarization, violence, hostility, torture, abuse of political power, corruption, alcoholism, drug addiction, sexual promiscuity and economic chaos.

One of the major obstacles to this much needed awareness seems to be that by and large our lives are so intensely self-affirming that we cannot see the forest for the trees. We are so accustomed to consider self-affirming behavior a law of nature, a self-evident matter, that we find it exceedingly difficult to look at affirmation in any other way than of *doing* something— whether for self or others. Rollo May's discourse on this subject is a prime example of this—we have commented on this already in *Born Only Once*. So is the current interest in promoting various methods of self-assertion by persons who have "discovered" the difference between assertion and aggression. These advocates do not seem to realize that the results of their methods can only be relative, and never touch the heart of the matter. For *effectivity* resulting from will-training, instead of being born in and from the person's *affectivity*, is nothing but another form of self-affirmation. This affective being-in-the-world, however, cannot be developed by training; it requires for its development the authentic affirmation by another, already affirmed person.

In other words, although it is true that shy, self-effacing, others-pleasing people can benefit from learning more assertive behavior, it must be realized that such training amounts to nothing more than helping the fearful unaffirmed person to do what the constitutionally more courageous, perhaps more talented, unaffirmed person does spontaneously: affirm himself. The end result of such training therefore is simply the replacing of one form of unhappy existence by another. This is one example of the need for professionals and paraprofessionals to be familiar with the meaning of affirmation. This, of course, is most easily learned from a clinical study of a human being who early in life is deprived of affirmation, the subject matter of this book.

Perhaps the best evidence for the existence of a fundamental difference between affirmation and self-affirmation is the present popularity of transcendental meditation and related efforts to escape from the unrest, tensions and frustrations of our much too busy world. It has been clearly demonstrated by clinical and laboratory testing that in these TM devotees the mental unrest gives way to calm, muscular tension to relaxation, beta waves to alpha waves, while hypertensives benefit from a reduction of their blood pressure. It is precisely these and other subjective and objective conditions of well-being which are spontaneously experienced and manifested by the adequately affirmed person, the person who is open to and finds delight in all existing good, and thus possesses what the restlessly striving, self-affirming person will never find.

This search for higher, more satisfying human values by so

many people and their finding them to a certain extent in transcendental meditation could easily lead too far. It might conceivably precipitate a violent rebellion against the utilitarian establishment and institutional churches, who must bear much of the responsibility for mankind's present unaffirmed state. This would be unfortunate since the establishment and the churches, too, are victims of self-affirmation. Instead of their rejection and overthrow they, too, must be aided to benefit from what has been learned about the psychological causes for self-affirming behavior and its detrimental effects on man and society. Modern man's search for inner peace and calm, in TM or otherwise, represents an instinctive attempt to reestablish a sound relationship between disordered, or better, reversed psychological processes, an attempt to correct the pathological dominance and emphasis accorded man's utility appetite over his pleasure appetite, his state of *effectivity* over that of *affectivity*, his self-affirmation over affirmation by others, his *doing* over his *being*. Why man has done this to himself and others over the ages is another question. The answer is not limited to the subject of affirmation, even though it is one of the most important facets.

Unfortunately, neither *Loving and Curing the Neurotic*[2] published in 1962, nor this book, provided an adequate opportunity to present much more than the personal clinical aspects of this dis-ease of modern man, and its contagious effects on his immediate milieu of family and community. In preparing the manuscript for this book, we realized that we had to be realistic in gauging the impact of our earlier writings on the psychiatric profession, the human sciences, and the general public. This impact is still a limited one, at least in the English speaking countries. Unless this syndrome is generally recognized in all its clinical and subclinical manifestations, together with its direct and indirect, overt and hidden effects on society, we will not be in a position to stem the tide of its increasingly destructive consequences on mankind. We intend to elaborate on this topic in future publications insofar as they have not yet already been covered in some of our monographs and books published in the

Netherlands or the United States of America in the past several years.

## MAN'S BASIC NEEDS: *Affirmation, Food, Shelter and Clothing*

All we want to state here is that we are convinced that without an anthropology based on the recognition of affirmation as a fundamental human need, to be mentioned in one breath with those for food, shelter and clothing, most current worldwide problems will defy solution. Here we do not hesitate to include such grave problems as pollution and depletion of natural resources, monetary chaos and self-destroying economies, rising crime and suicide rates, overpopulation and abortion, war and peace, development of new nations and the survival of others.

We would like to add that we cannot but feel optimistic about the eventual outcome of future efforts to deal with those critical situations once they are recognized to have been caused and perpetuated by self-affirming individuals. Many years of clinical experience have revealed to us tremendous creative, life-giving forces which emanate from authentic affirmation. For example, when *affectivity*, rather than *effectivity*, characterizes the life style and attitudes of affirmed men and women, they actually experience a *need* to have fewer material goods in order to live in quiet joy and inner peace. If this is true, then it is to be expected that a more affirmed and affirming population will show a much greater readiness toward equal distribution of goods among nations, than can be expected from an unaffirmed population that must be prodded by moral exhortation, if not by threat or force, by its rulers.

Likewise, in trying to prevent a much-feared population explosion current controversial, if not immoral, approaches, necessary in largely self-affirming populations, can be avoided when affirmed leaders govern affirmed citizens. Affirmed and affirming individuals actually find their deepest joy and satisfaction in exercising self-restraint—in all areas, the sexual one included—when their reason or the happiness of others require this.

Our optimism is further enhanced by the immediate recognition and widespread reception accorded our views by the man in the street this past decade. In the Netherlands our books, lectures, and radio and TV presentations on the subject of affirmation, have brought thousands of letters and hundreds of requests for personal appearances and consultations. Underlying these responses is an intense discontent with prevailing conditions of existence and relating, and a universal hunger for authentic happiness and love. This in a sector of the world where people have everything, where a socialistic government tries to satisfy every need from the cradle to the grave, and people do pretty well as they please with minimal attention to moral laws!

The professional world, on the other hand, has been much slower and more hesitant to respond to our interpretations and conclusions derived from our observations in clinical practice. This is not surprising as they touch upon matters not taught or discussed in medical schools: man's relationship to his Creator, the nature of his happiness, rational psychology, and so on. However, the tide seems to be turning. The crucial distinction between affirmation and self-affirmation is being recognized by an increasing number of our colleagues. Perhaps the main credit for this should go to Dr. J.J.G. Prick, Professor of Neurology and Psychiatry at the Catholic University of Nijmegen and adviser to the World Health Organization. In 1973 he published a monograph entitled: *The Significance of the Work of Dr. A.A.A. Terruwe for Psychiatry*, in which he wrote, "In addition to Dr. Terruwe's discovery of the frustration (deprivation) neurosis, its proper placement in the diagnostic classification of psychiatric disorders, the development of a corresponding form of psychotherapy based on the process of affirmation, she also contributed significantly to the field of preventive medicine or orthopedagogy...."

We are also happy to add that in recent years some leaders in government, church, military establishment, health organizations, labor unions and schools of economy, have contacted us for the purpose of investigating in what manner our insights can serve their desire and obligation to better the lives of the people entrusted to their care and guidance. Several related their frustrations about the practical ineffectiveness of what otherwise seemed to be sound theories of management and leadership, even when taking into consideration man's psychological limitations. These considerations, we advised them, were based on the brilliant clinical discoveries of Sigmund Freud, but did not encompass those of the unaffirmed state, which simply do not respond to psychoanalytic therapies, behavior modification, drug therapy and the like. We have assured them that they can expect far superior results for their efforts when they, too, come to realize that much in our sick society in some way or other is caused or aggravated by self-affirmation.

We invite further exchanges of ideas with anyone who shares our confidence and hope that the sad state of world affairs can be made a thing of the past by respecting all of man's fundamental needs, not only those of food, shelter and clothing. For some time we have been convinced that the man in the street must become an active part of the psychiatric team, of any healing efforts aimed at the wholeness of the human being. But this will not be enough—the *leaders* in our society must be involved too. Since it is essential that our leaders are not self-affirming individuals we must make every effort to ensure that only affirmed and affirming persons are elected and appointed to the most responsible positions in government, church, universities, business, labor unions, communications media, and so on!

1—*The Neurosis in the Light of Rational Psychology,* A.A.A. Terruwe, M.D., translated by C.W. Baars, M.D.; P.J. Kenedy & Sons, New York, 1960.

2—A.A.A. Terruwe, M.D. and C.W. Baars, M.D., Arlington House Publishers, New Rochelle, N. Y.

# BIBLIOGRAPHY

Adler, Mortimer, J. *The Time of Our Lives*. New York: Holt, Rinehart & Winston, 1970.

    *The Idea of Freedom*. Garden City: Doubleday, Vol. I, 1958, Vol. II, 1961.

Aquinas, Thomas. *Summa Theologica*. 3 vols., New York: Benziger Bros., 1947.

    *Commentary on Nichomachean Ethics*.

Aristotle. *Nichomachean Ethics*.

Arnold, Magda B. *Emotion and Personality*, 2 vols., New York: Columbia University Press, 1960.

Baars, Conrad W. *Born Only Once*. Franciscan Herald Press, Chicago, Ill., 1975.

    "Christian Anthropology of Thomas Aquinas," *The Priest*, October, 1974.

    *Sex, Love and the Life of the Spirit*. Chicago: Priory Press, 1966.

    *The Psychology of Obedience*. St. Louis: B. Herder Book Co., 1965.

    "Thomas Aquinas and the Cure of Obsessive-Compulsive Neurotics" in *The Catholic Doctor in Changing Societies*, Vol. I., London, 1962.

Boekel, C. W. Van. *Katharsis*. Utrecht: DeFontein, 1957.

Boxtel, J. P. Van. "Moraal en Affectiviteit" in *De Menselyke Persoon in de christelyke moraal*, 1958.

    "Moraal en Gevoelsleven volgens Thomas van Aquino" in *Tydschrift voor Philosophie*, June, 1959.

Brennan, Robert E. *General Psychology*. New York: Macmillan, 1937.

    *Thomistic Psychology*. New York: Macmillan, 1941.

Calon, P. J. A. *De Jongen*. Haarlem: De Toorts, 1958.

    "Ontwikkeling van de menselyke persoon. Consequenties voor de christelyke moraal." *Voordracht gehouden op studiedagen voor de priesters van het aartsbisdom Utrecht en bisdom Groningen*. August, 1958.

    and Prick, J. J. G. *Psychologische Grondbegrippen*.

Donceel, J. F. *Philosophical Psychology*. New York: Sheed and Ward, 1955.

Duynstee, W. J. A. J. *Verspreide Opstellen*. Roermond-Maaseik: J. J. Romen & Zonen, 1963.

Ford, John C. *Depth Psychology, Morality and Alcoholism*. Weston, Mass.: Weston College, 1951.

and Gerald Kelly, S.J. *Contemporary Moral Theology*, Vols. I and II, Westminster, Md., The Newman Press, 1959.

Freud, Sigmund, *A General Introduction to Psychoanalysis*. Garden City: Garden City Publishing Co., 1943.

Gerets, J. P. *Psychasthenie en frustratie neurose.*

Graauw, H.J.M. de. *Een Academische Opleiding in De Pedagogiek*. Nymegen, 1972.

Guardini, Romano. *The End of the Modern World*. New York: Sheed & Ward, 1956.

    *Das Gute, das Gewissen und die Sammlung*. Mainz: Matthias-Grunewald-Verlag.

Journet, Charles. *The Meaning of Evil*. New York: P. J. Kenedy & Sons, 1963.

Joyce, Mary Rosera. *Love Responds to Life—The Challenge of Humanae Vitae*, Prow, 1971.

    and Joyce, Robert E. *New Dynamics in Sexual Love*. Collegeville, Minn.: St. John's University Press, 1970.

Kelsey, Morton. *Healing and Christianity*. New York: Harper & Row, 1973.

Kuhlman, Kathryn. *I Believe in Miracles*. Englewood Cliffs, N. J.: Prentice-Hall, 1969.

MacNutt, Francis, O.P. *Healing*. Notre Dame, Ind.: Ave Maria Press, 1974.

Meany, John. "Reflections on Thomism and Client-Centered Psychotherapy." Paper presented at the 16th Annual Scientific Session, Guild of Catholic Psychiatrists. Los Angeles, 1964.

Noyes, Arthur P. and Kolb, Lawrence C. *Modern Clinical Psychiatry*. Philadelphia: W.B. Saunders Co., 1963.

Pfürtner, Stephanus. *Triebleben und Sittliche Vollendung*. Freiburg, Schweiz: Universitätsverlag, 1958.

Pieper, Josef. *Fortitude and Temperance*. New York: Pantheon Books, 1954.

    *Happiness and Contemplation*. New York: Pantheon Books, 1958.

    *Leisure—The Basis of Culture*. New York: Pantheon Books, 1952.

Rahner, Hugo. *Man at Play*. New York: Herder and Herder, 1967.

Royo, Antonio, and Aumann, Jordan. *The Theology of Christian Perfection*. Dubuque: Priory Press, 1962.

Rzadkiewicz, Arnold L. *The Philosophical Bases of Human Liberty According to Thomas Aquinas*. Washington, D. C.: Catholic University Press, 1949.

Sanford, Agnes. *The Healing Gifts of the Spirit*. Philadelphia: J. B. Lippincott Co., 1966.

Shlemon, Barbara Leahy. *Healing Prayer*. Notre Dame, Ind.: Ave Maria Press, 1976.

Smith, Vincent Edward. *The General Science of Nature*. Milwaukee: Bruce Books, 1958.

Terruwe, Anna A. *De Frustratie neurose*. Roermond-Masseik: Romen & Zonen. 1962.

    *De liefde bouwt een woning*. Roermond-Maaseik: Romen & Zonen.

    *Emotional Growth in Marriage*. Paramus, N. J.: Paulist Press, 1968.

*Geloven zonder angst en vrees.* Roermond-Masseik: Romen & Zonen, 1969.

*The Neurosis in the Light of Rational Psychology*—translated by C. W. Baars, M.D. New York: P. J. Kenedy & Sons, 1960.

*Opening van zaken.* In usum privatum. Nymegen, 1964.

*Psychopathic Personality and Neurosis.* translated by C. W. Baars, M.D. New York: P. J. Kenedy & Sons, 1958.

Tournier, Paul. *The Person Reborn.* New York: Harper & Row, 1966.

Vann, Gerald. *The Heart of Man.* London: Longmans, Green & Co., 1945.

*Morals and Man.* New York: Sheed and Ward, 1960.

Wilhelmsen, Frederick D. *The Metaphysics of Love.* New York: Sheed & Ward, 1962.

# INDEX